Vajramuktiyoga

Zen & Martial arts.. probing in deeper subtle worlds

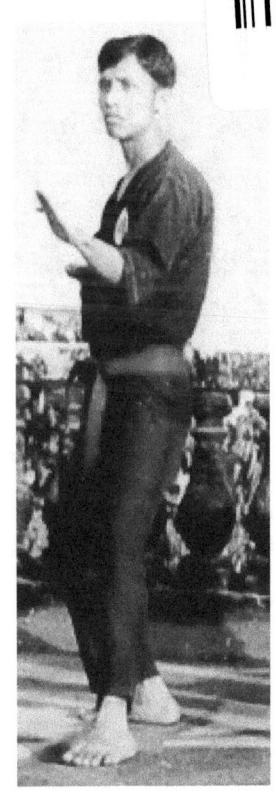

*This book is dedicated to Perfect Master
Lord Anami*

*Honest readers! I beseech you with folded
hands to*

*Favor this book with intuitive awareness &
be helpful*

To others to give birth to their own ideas

For seeing live in channel http://youtube.com/c/DrChandraSkeekhar

www.ulslab.blogspot.com

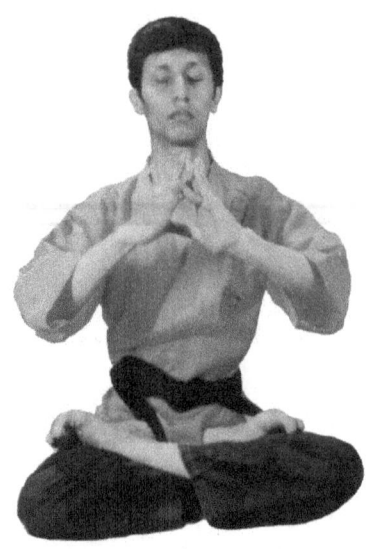

GLOSSARY OF SANSKRIT TERMS

1) Aashirwaad Blessing.
2) Abhyasa   Practice.
3) Abhinivesah Instinctive clinging to life or fear of death
4) Adhara   A support.
5) Agama   Evidence of an acceptable authority.
6) Ahamkara   Ego.
7) Ahimsa   Non-violence.
8) Ajna-chakra   situated between the

                          Eyebrows
9) Alasya   Idleness, lazyness.

10) Anahata-chakra   the chakra situated in the cardiac region.

11) Anga   the part.

12) Anumana   An inference.

13) Antar   Inside.

14) Apana   Vital air which controls the function of elimination of faeces.

15) Ardha   Half.

16) Astanga   Eight parts of the Yoga.

17) Asana   Posture.

18) Asta   Eight.

19) Asmita   "I"ness or Egotism.

20) Asteya   Non-stealing.

21) Asvini-mudra the contraction of the anal sphincter.

22) Atma   Soul.

23) Aum   the primordial
sound.
24) Avidhya   Ignorance.
25) Avastha   State.
26) Ayurveda   Traditional Indian
system of medicine.
27) Bandha   In a posture where
                certain parts of the
                body are
                contracted or
                locked or
                controlled.
28) Bahya   Outside.
29) Bhastrika   Pranayam where
air is forcibly draw in &
    out as bellows used in a
furnace.
30) Bhoga   Enjoyment.
31) Bhramari   Pranayama where
                during exhalation a

soft   humming
sound like the
murmuring of a
bee is made

32) Bhrumadhya the place
    between the eyebrows.
33) Bhujangasana   Cobra poses
or posture.
34) Brahama randhra- an aperture
in the crown of the
                    Head
35) Chakra   Centre of vital
              channels in the
              etheric body.
36) Chandra   Moon.
37) Chakrasana the wheel posture.
38) Chitta   Consciousness.
39) Darshan   Sight of a guru or
deity.

40) Dhyana   Meditation.

41) Dharana   Complete attention.

42) Dhanurasana Bow posture.

43) Dukha   Sorrow.

44) Dvesha   Hate or dislike.

45) Eka   One.

46) Ekagrata   concentration

47) Eka pada   one leg.

48) Gow mudra Cow posture.

49) Guru   Dispeller of the darkness.

50) Guna   Constituents of nature.

51) Hatha Yoga 'Ha' means the sun and 'tha' means the moon. Hatha Yoga is to harmonize   the

solar and lunar
energy.

52) Hanumanasana   Posture
named after Hanumana.

53) Halasana   the plough poses.
54) Indriyas   Sense organs.
55) Isvara or Eshvana God.
56) Jalandhara bandha   Chin
Lock.
57) Janu   the knee.
58) Janusirsasana   the posture
where head
touches to
the knee.
59) Japa   the repetation of
the Mantra.
60) Jivatma   the individual soul.
61) Jnana   Knowledge.
62 Kaivalya   bliss

63) Kapalabhati   Forehead brightener.

64) Karmendriya Organs of action hands, feet's and speech.

65) Khandharasana   the shoulder poses.

66) Kriya Yoga- higher yogic science

67) Kumbhak   Retention.

68) Kundalini   the serpent power coiled

69) Lobha   Greed.

70) Makar   A crocodile.

71) Makarasana-the pose resembling crocodile.

72) Mana   Mind.

73) Manipura Chakra-the chakra situated in the

region of the
naval.

74) Matsyendrasana   Spinal twist
pose, named after
   Matsyendranath.

75) Mayurasana- the peacock
poses.

76) Matsyasana- the fish pose.

77) Moola   Root.

78) Moha   Attachment.

79) Moksha   Liberation.

80) Mrdu   mild.

81) Mudra   A sealing posture.

82) Muladhara Chakra   the
                   chakra situated
                   in the pelvis,
                   above the
                      anus, at the
                   root of the spine.

83) Nabhi   Naval.

84) Nadis   Subtle channels.
85) Nauli   A process in which
the abdominal muscles   are
moved from one side to the
other in a surging motion.
86) Nirodha   Dissolution.
87) Niyama   Rules of
Obervance.
88) Parmatma   the Supreme Soul.
89) Parivrtta   Turned around.
90) Parsva   Side.
91) Paschimottana   Intense
                   stretch of the back
                   side of the body
                    from the heels.
92) Prajna   Wisdom.
93) Prakriti   Nature.

94) Prana   Vital breath.

95) Pranayama Control of breath.
96) Pratyahara Withdrawl of the mind from senses.
97) Punya   Virtue.
98) Rajas   One of the three gunas, quality of the nature known as activity.
99) Rechaka   Exhalation or expirtaion.
100) Sadhana   Practice
101) Sadhaka   An aspirant
102) Samana   One of the five pranas
103) Somsaya   Doubt
104) Samskara Impressions of the past
105) Sanatana an eternal path
106) Santosa   Contentment
107) Sarvanga the whole body

108) Sattva   One of the three
             gunas of the nature
109) Shalbhasana The locust pose
or posture.
110) Sirsha   the head
111) Smrti   Memory
112) Sraddha   Faith
113) Sukhasana -the easy pose
114) Suddhi kriya -the cleansing
process
115) Supta   Sleeping
116) Surya   the sun
117) Sunya   Void
118) Sushumna -the vital channel
                situated inside the
                spinal column
119) Surya Namaskar-Salutations
to the sun
120) Svadhisthana Chakra-   the
                chakra situated

	above the organs of generation
121) Svadhyaya	Self study
122) Tada	A mountaion
123) Tapah	Austerity
124) Tamas	One of the three gunas of the nature known as darkness
125) Tadagi	Lake
126) Trikona	Triangle pose

CONTENTS

ACKNOWLEDGMENTS

I Acknowledge and respect the genius of all those who had touched my being and we happen to exchange our views globally. It is impossible to mention the names of all philosophers. Scientists, performing artists, workers from all walks of life, who have become instrumental in helping this name and form named shekhar, grow to know the formless.

I am obliged to the members of my advisory Committee especially to Dr H N mistry and Dr Pradeep kumar Biswasfor their helpful suggestions Pradeep kumar Chief editor Indian express for valuable advice to be helpful by making human beings aware and presenting the awareness to the public. To Pratap Antony, Pradeep kumar, Pradeep kamat, Vijayrane, Basel Hoshidaruwalla, Darshana doshi and Manibhai doshi close associate of Shri Subash Chandra Bose and Founder of Rotary clubs chain at South Bombay.Late Rami chand Rajbar, Mani chand Rajbar from Chand Dynasty, for giving help and inspiration. A Hillman from navy named Pathak, Bhaskar Prasad Gildhiyal.Arun pradhan and family, Ujjwal Roy, Mahesh jabbar. A Chinese friend and fellow practitioner Yu Chu Liang who helped vajramukti grow. My friends and students who worked for the growth and increasing the awareness of the people, who happen to come in touch with me. These were my friend Unnikrishnan Nair, Bimal kumar choubey, Surendra singhRawat, James,Richard,AbhisekhGhosh,Sha un cooper,Sheffy George, Rajat pandey.Ryan Cooper, Kamlesh Mishra, Sumeet kumar.

It gives me a great feeling of contentment by remembering my student Dr Ajey Dambal from Stanford University from United States. I taught him little of vajramukti and he could remove all other thoughts and concentrate on one thought

Words are inappropriate to thank my wife Shobha bhatt without her support it was not possible.

I don't know how to thank Dr Ram Bhosle descendent of Chattrapati Shivaji Raja Bhosle and student of Sir Herbert

Barker of United Kingdom, with whom I spent many years in awakening.

AUTHORS NOTE

What led me to coin this term Vajramukti I had studied in books of metaphysics that human body is a miniature cosmos. All religions and philosophies speak about inner light and inner sound. Yogic sciences speak about soundless sound. One evening after meditation I lied down, with a thud or a jerk I was inside my body. My body became as big as universe. I could feel the gigantic roaring of the planets and sound of whole cosmos inside my being. I could feel every chakra inside my body as given in Yogic sciences. Many such experiences and study of philosophy sitting at the lap of Dr Ram Bhosle student of Sir Herbert barker of United Kingdom came into my awareness. My Martial arts teachers Sensai Oliver Fernandez and Sensai Leslie Fernandez and yoga teachers Dilip sir, Alka Tai, Usha Tai, Bapu saheb and Doctors from conventional and unconventional world helped me grow this art of martial way with yoga of healing known as

Vajramuktiyoga

INTRODUCTION

All dramas, Novels, books of natural sciences are written or presented in a process of making human beings more aware. I am presenting my awareness by means of this book. I would be highly obliged if this book serves as the means, In the process of understanding the universality of the spirit.

What is the process involved in making human being more aware? How to get rid of conditioning and live from instant to instant: from second to second?

Vajramukti is one such technique. By practicing Vajramukti accumulation of venous blood is controlled. The body is filled with abundant energy. The brain centers and spinal cord are strengthened. Memory is improved. It prevents the decay of the tissues, increases the life force. It is condensed with kriya yoga,laya yoga, nada yoga and Hatha yoga in conjunction with Martial arts and meditation. It may be recalled that in the days of Bodhidharma Martial arts was not separated from meditation. In the present day world however, the two are poles apart or at least that is what the lay man gathers. Most people think that Buddha and Bodhidharma are the same.Bodhidharma was a totally different action enshrined personality. He was the man responsible for spreading Martial arts from India to China. He went from India to China to spread the messages of Buddhism. He was born as a prince in south part of

India. He renounced the kingdom in search of truth. It is believed that when he intended to leave China, for the Himalayas, at the same night he was poisoned by some rivals and they buried him. After three years he was found by someone known to him.

He was with his staff in his hand and one of his sandals dangling on his staff. Bodhidharma said to that man; just inform my people that I am going to going to Himalayas forever.

When the man reached there, they all opened the tomb. To their surprise, one sandal was still there.

Vajramukti meaning from action to liberation Vajramukti gives laymen an awareness of what it is to meditate and keep oneself fighting fit. Martial arts are not for street fighting. Street fighting can be learnt from any roadside thug. Martial art is for coordination of mind and body.

When you are angry you start clinging with anger, because of this anger some chemicals are released in your blood. The situation is created. It puts you in a state either to fight or not to fight. If this dilution of power of mind through the entity anger is controlled wonders can be done. Your all body processes follow your mind. If your mind interprets someone as your friend or enemy, the body follows accordingly. But when for you there is no friend or enemy, and then there is the higher path. Then the awareness expands.

Vajramukti is a non violent art uses body and its processes as means towards an end to know thyself and holistic healing. I am trying to describe or put my awareness of nonviolence, by quoting dialogue between Yulteshwar giri and Paramhansa Yogananda author of Autobiography of a Yogi.

Yukteshwarji was interpreting the ancient texts.

Yoganandaji was also sitting there. A mosquito sat upon his thigh and was distracting his attention. Yogananda raised his hand, but at the same time he remembered Patanjalis sutra of nonviolence {ahimsa}.

"Why didn't you finish the job?" said Yukteshwarji.

"MasterDo you advocate taking life?"

Replied Yoganandaji"No, but in your mind you had already struck the death blow.

"I don't understand"

"By ahimsa Patanjali meant
removal of the desire to kill"

This world is conveniently arranged
for a literal practice of ahimsa.
Man may be compelled to
exterminate harmful creatures; he
is not under a similar compulsion
to feel anger or animosity.

Patanjali yoga sutra 11...35 says.

"In the presence of a man
perfected in ahimsa {nonviolence}

Enmity does not arise."

One can talk about nonviolence,
but deep inside violence is still

present and it can erupt anytime.

It is easy for the masters to practice non-violence because they are totally aware. But not for everyone, so one has to be alert all the time in order to increase his awareness.

There are still infinite numbers of paths to be explored and this may lead us to several new and delightful phenomena.

One can spend a lifetime exploring, but the purpose is not served by mere exploration. It is a question of opening up new avenues. One such avenue is Vajramukti.

It is a technique which combines skills of martial arts, yoga and meditation. It is an integrated approach to one's self improvement and inner development.

Vajramukti when it put into practice not only serves the purpose of refining the mind and body culture but also encourages you to think beyond the realms of awareness or seek greener pastures.

I am sure you would have heard of umpteen numbers of techniques like transcendental meditation{TM}auto suggestion to control the mind Hypnosis etc.But Vajramukti is unique in the sense that it uses no short cut.

It calls for investment of your valuable time as attention. It also awaits your willingness to understand and grasp new ideas.

In short there is something to be had, but not an ice-cream on the platter: for it has to be chewed or assimilated over the years.

Now the question arises, why pick on Vajramukti? Why turn away from the shortcuts or spend time with an entirely new concept? The answer lies in the text penned by

Dr Chandra Shekhar Bhatt, who has painstakingly compiled experiences theories or solutions to several key issues that have time and again bogged the human mind.

Yoga and Martial Art are not opposed to one another but on the contrary they have the same origin and are complementary to each other. It was from Swami Chakrajit & Dr. Ram Bhosle that I learnt that Yoga is the base of all Martial Arts. I came out with a new avenue called Vajramukti that was my first book released at Mumbai. It was very nicely read and understood by shaolin society of United kingdom and they had put it in their site which was really good study on Vajramukti so I am giving those words here..A BRIEF HISTORY OF KUNG FU YOGA Yoga has captured the attention of the West as the latest fashion. Celebrities such as Sting, Woody Harrelson and the Grateful Dead have made it part of their practice. Even Madonna attributes her latest incarnation (albeit sacrilegiously) to yoga. And just the aerobics craze found new life by fusing with martial arts and jazz dance; martial arts have also begun making some similar trendy fusions to yoga. Not only are many martial artists practicing Yoga as cross training, new hybrids are being born out of the imaginations of both savvy salespeople and sloppy translators. Taoist Yoga, even Shaolin Yoga, has begun to emerge as the new thing on the health scene and in the martial circles. But what is Yoga exactly and how does it relate to martial arts? Most Westerners only think of Yoga as extreme contortionist-like stretching in truth, it is a much more profound discipline than most of those fad followers believe. Yoga is a time- honored method of self-realization than may even be the very root of martial arts The word 'Yoga' comes from the same root as the word 'yoke' and it is documented as early as 2000 BCE. What most people envision as Yoga, those contortionist postures, is really only one small aspect of a much larger field of practices. Those postures are called 'Asana' which translates as 'seat'. According to the Yoga Sutras of Patanjali the fundamental text of Yoga by the 'father' of Yoga Asana is the third 'limb' of an eightfold path known as 'Astanga'. The other seven limbs are Yama (observance of morals), Niyama (self-restraint), Pranayama (breath control), Pratyahara (sense inhibition), Dharana (concentration), Dhyana (meditation) and Samadhi (ecstasy). Beyond this, there are many other forms of Yoga, such as Karma Yoga, which is sort of like a discipline devoted to doing good deeds. Essentially, Yoga embodies a wide variety of disciplines that are vehicles for spiritual transformation. Generalizing Yoga to Asana alone is just as shallow as generalizing all martial arts to breaking boards alone. However this generalization persists in the West for the same reason breaking boards persists- it is spectacular media image of these ancient arts. This misconception muddles the creation myths of our own beloved martial arts. According to popular legend, Bodhidharma brought the direct lineage of Buddhism to China from India in 526 BCE. He arrived at Shaolin Temple in Honan, and founded Shaolin Kung Fu and Zen Buddhism (known as Chan in Chinese). This is the most common creation myth in martial arts, since Shaolin Kung Fu is also the root of main Japanese and Korean styles. Only three forms comprised Bodhidharma Shaolin Kung Fu muscle tendon change (Yijinging), bone marrow washing (Xisuijing) and the 18 Arhats palm (Luohanshibazhang), only the third form was martial the first two were Qigong forms. Since Bodhidharma was Indian, many sources postulate that he based his Shaolin Kung Fu upon Yoga. The postures of Yoga Asana do bear a striking resemblance to postures' of Qigong, so much so, that one cannot help but wonder.

Was there a connection between Yoga and KungFu? The answer is very confusing. As previously mentioned Yoga Asana, is only one aspect of Yoga. Many martial scholars make common mistake of inferring Bodhidharma's teachings were based on Yoga because Yoga Asana resembles Qigong. This is a little misleading. Some Yoga scholars do not believe that many Asana (at least those postures that resemble Qigong) were even around at the time of Bodhidharma. The only Asana that can be confirmed archeologically is padmasana, or 'seated lotus' position. This pose is fundamental in many meditation practices. Indeed, Bodhidharma was most famous for his practice of sitting meditation. According to legend he sat meditating on a rock for nine years. Sitting meditation is the cornerstone of his innovation of Buddhism, Zen. In fact, he invented Shaolin Kung Fu because he felt that the monks of Shaolin who were too weak to endure the hardship of prolonged meditation, So if lotus was the only asana of Bodhidharma's time and if he did incorporate it into his new Kung Fu practice, it might be said that

Shaolin Kung Fu was based on Yoga Asana. This is still based on a lot of assumptions, but at least the terminology is more accurate. A more intriguing theory is that Bodhidharma based Shaolin Kung Fu Pranayama. Pranayama is the fourth limb of Patanjali's Yoga. Like Qigong, Pranayama refers to the exercises that cultivate the life force that resides in the breath. This concept alienates most Western post- Descartean thinkers; our worldview separates mind and body. A life force that resides in the breath has no place here. Breath is body and life force is mind. The idea of something that is both upsets our dominant paradigm. However, the ancient Greeks had shared this breath life-force philosophy of the Indians and the Chinese. They called it Pneuma. This is the same root word from where we get 'pneumonia'. Language fossils of this idea are more evident from the Latin root word 'spirare'. This is where we get the words 'spirit' and 'respiration'. The link between breath and life force is clearly seen in words like 'inspiration', 'expiration', and 'aspiration'. More subtle examples exists in terms like'conspiracy', which can be interpreted as both 'to breathe together' as well as 'to share the same spirit.' By embracing these ancient philosophies, mind and body can be reunited and Qi (or Prana or Pneuma) becomes more comprehensible. Ironically, some translators have chosen to call Qigong 'Taost Yoga'. English has its limitation. We have no words for Qigong or Yoga in English. The advantage of English is that we can just adopt these words from their original language. While 'Taoist Yoga' might appeal to some new age marketers, it is kind of like calling instant ramen noodles-'Buddhist spaghetti', It is confusing enough without scrambling terms. Qigong in China predates Bodhidharma by several centuries. Even if he added Yoga Pranayama to his two forms of Qigong, the results are undistinguishable. While Bodhidharma's Qigong methods are elegant, Qigong has long standing precedents that surpass his contributions. So if neither the physical poses of Asana, nor the breath control method of Pranayama which contribute to the movements of Bodhidharma's Qigong, can we still say that KungFu find its roots in Yoga? The answer lies in the seventh limb of Patanjali's eightfold path- Dhyana (meditation) both of the terms Zen (short for Zenna) and Chan (short for Channa) were phonetic translation of Dhyana. This was the soul of Bodhidharma's contributions. He infused meditation into martial practice. Common sense, backed with archaeological evidence, clearly show that martial practices existed in China previous to Bodhidharma. So why

Bodhidharma is even credited as the founder of Kung Fu it was his introduction of meditation to martial arts that revealed the heart of Yoga spiritual transformation. Bodhidharma elevated martial skills into a vehicle for spiritual transformation. He put the 'art' into martial arts. On this level, martial arts became just as B.K.S Iyengar says, 'It is like Yoga' Before Bodhidharma, martial arts were just a means of self-defense. Today, in his wake, it can become a method of self-realization. Today, it is easy to lose sight of the spiritual especially in the martial arts. Each day brings another deluge of information overload, stressing our attention to its breaking point, and jamming our ability to focus on the clear pursuit of the way. We get defensive. We forget Bodhidharma's teachings. Right now, many new practitioners completely disregard any notion of spirituality. Eager to ride coattails of the latest fashion trends, Kung Fu and Yoga have become strange bedfellows in today's health clubs. It is a strange twist, perhaps another repercussion of our mind-body worldview, which has placed these two venerated vehicles for spiritual transformation in our gymnasiums of physical transformation. From out of China's Wushu Guan and India's Yoga Ashrams and the shimmering silks and diaphanous cottons of the master of old now it's all spandex and logos. No more burning incense to honor our ancestors Bodhidharma and Patanjali. In fact, a few health club practitioners even know who these seminal figures are. Instead it is the latest exercise machines and boon boxes. The health clubs tend to greatly simplify the disciplines to give them the wildest appeal. Yoga is often reduced to the Asana alone just as martial arts are often reduced to only aerobic kicking and punching. The deeper meanings beneath the underlying philosophies are usually lost. While many of today's instructors struggle to maintain an air of tradition in their health club classrooms, the main marketing motivation for many of those clubs is the vain pursuit of a higher butt. While this might be a supplementary bonus, imagine Bodhidharma's reaction. This is most evident in cross training. Yoga is said to compliment martial arts and vice versa. In its actuality, both Yoga and martial arts are complete systems. Study either one thoroughly and there is no need of anything else. The concept of complimentary training implies that there is a deficit. But after a thousand of years of research and development, neither Yoga nor Kung Fu has any gaps to be filled. Both disciplines offer a fulfilling lifetime quest; all that need be done is that you pursue it for a lifetime. It is only our MTV- driven attention span that makes us move to the next thing before truly engaging the previous one. There have been some hybrids of Kung Fu and Yoga like 'Shaolin Yoga' designed to catch our attention with the promise of filling the two 'needs' at once. For the most part, these mongrel schools are really marketing ploys, not actual innovation. Both compound the issue. As a matter of fact, there is already an eastern fusion of yoga to martial arts that completely omits bodhidharma. the modern indian master chandra shekhar bhatt is an exponent of a hybrid of martial arts and yoga known as v a j r a m u k t i he has had enough of a following to publish books, but you would have to go all the way to bombay to train with him. Despite these criticisms, this new popularity actually reflects upon both disciplines, because now they are available to a greater population. While health clubs are far from ideal settings to study either Kung Fu or Yoga, they are better than not studying at all. And many of those new converts may eventually seek to fill the spiritual vacuum by pursuing the arts on a deeper level. The next generation of traditional practitioners when the facts die down, a fraction of those followers will undoubtedly remain to join our martial community more seriously. Growth, expansion, Empowerment- we are all seeking some sort of transformation. Whether it is the elusive feeling of security of crime ridden streets, or the shedding of a few unwanted pounds, or even the pursuit of spiritual ecstasy, we are all on our own personal quest. We choose the ancient paths as a means of transformation to these transformations. And yet, these ancient paths are modern incarnations that must grapple with modern misconceptions. Martial arts are built on the insecurity and paranoia of violence. We can easily slide into a combat mode; after all, it is hard to be spiritual when someone is kicking you in the head. But that spiritual aspect remains for those who wish to pursue it. Yoga is unencumbered with the burden of violence, so its means misconceptions too, they are not as pronounced as ours are. Almost

15 centuries ago, Yoga offered the martial arts to self-realization. The door is still open. but leave your boom box behindI am deeply indebted to India's renowned spiritual artist Sadhak Shivanand Saraswati and all these great personalities who have guided me and helped me in one way or other in my research & search for truth and perfection. In brief if I would define Vajramukti or Indian martial arts philosophy it would be with following words.

Accepting all ways as the way as ancient Indians has accepted all religions even the one not accepted by western world the Parsis were accepted in this land of

Humans. Different martial arts are like different religions goal of all is same to go inside, once you start travelling inside there is no religion no path no way… when individuality is dissolved where are the tools to operate we also don't know how to give awareness of that to all

I saw a boy of eleven years attacked by some seven or eight people his bag of tomato was thrown he had no knowledge of martial art he just moved with whoever was nearby touching the empty space he found and went on with all and got away collecting his left over tomatoes. If you can move within the space by just observing you have made your martial art. But it's not possible with all if we are depressed due to various reasons may be we won't be able to defend all the time the only way is to train by inculcating your experiences and making your own system.

But if you cannot due to past imprints on your consciousness to what Hindus believe as karmas then you can go to some systems or learn from the event you pass through and make your own awareness system suiting you the best. As master Lee said if you understand the principals of different arts and if you learn to flow with the movements you have made the system for your body mind quantum, same as master lee worked on in the name of man who was once fluid.

Yoga the way of life given by the people who went inside and thought of helping people because in essence we are all spark of that same light. Hindu kings send their love sometime as accepting Buddhism and sending monks around the world to spread love they accepted Jews and others from world as their own extensions. Martial arts spreading were just the byproduct there were many arts remained silently flowing in its own accordance. If you don't like yoga as a Hindu word you can learn from the western people who learned yoga extensively and came out adding their awareness to it as Ida Rolfs system or her many students developing the branches in many forms, and if you find short of economic needs come in India there are still people who teach free, out of love but learn to relax and then be in your way until you feel need to know thyself.

History of Indian martial art is beyond time framework there are masters living in Himalayas who can attack you and change your thought process from thousands miles, but they don't because you are undivided part of the whole and you have your own free will. Once a professor of Harvard University asked Swami Vivekanandaji, whether he knew about anyone who has studied Self-Hypnosis? Swamiji said in western countries whatever they call as hypnotism, it is just the part of the actual text which Rishis called as—— atmapasammohan (dehypnotisation) they say, you are already hypnotized, you have to dehypnotize.

Yato vacho nivartante aprapt manasa sah

Anandam bramano vidvan na bibhate kadachan

With mind the speech, without knowing that, comes back,

By knowing that one, the fear remains not this is dehypnotisation.

Swami ji was not in favor of treating people by hypnotism. He said that every individual has power of Braham. By someone else controlling it, there are very much chances of you losing your own will power.

There are master livings of age more than two thousand years. Hindu kings Ashoka abandon martial arts because his being was touched so deeply by the adverse effects the war gives. Chinese have come to the land of ancient India at the time of Moriya dynasty, when Nalanda was the center of education in its natural sense and essence. Flowing in accordance with nature all subjects were unfolded in its natural way, understanding everything as spark of light from which all came into existence.

The science of Yoga is the base of Indian martial art which goes subtly and naturally beyond modern psycho-physiology for example while I was teaching yoga I came across a female with psychosomatic problem it took three years for her to become normal so as she don't know if she was facing such problem. In psycho systems they treat patients to eliminate emotions by relieving past experiences same is achieved by practicing one moola bandha of yogic sciences but it takes time to affect the centers at brain.

All ranks, all rules, all pre-orchestrated movement, all limitations are respected by us and carried forward as development of mind body relationship ,except for the limitation of mind and body is the way of moving from "Law of Nature" to beyond the juxtaposition of mind and body or mind and matter through meditation. Indian martial Art is a system of real education working as a bud transforms into flower no force required it's the relaxed way of Yoga. Meditation on third eye is the way wherein you can break the knot of mind and matter. Agastya muni had coded down these in the form of sutras for good people to read and practice through meditation but very few people can excel in that like Prakasan from south part of India could do that he could attack without contact within 10 feets and the person will be knocked down , Indian

Martial Art is a system beyond normal understanding because of its vast history wherever Hindu kings ruled around the world they never exploited the humanity inspite of such high knowledge on martial arts the king like Ashoka renounced weapons it was due to love for humanity understanding the higher purpose of being in the human birth. By reading the book by a yogi who left his body voluntarily at united states at a last speech uttering that where Ganges flow men leave their houses in search of god lo..my soul have touched that sod and he left the body can you imagine, have you ever noticed such happening. His book is named Autobiography of a yogi..... Let me tell you about the interest on yoga in RUSSIA, Justice V. R Krishna Iyer former judge of Supreme Court of India, at the time of visiting a town near Leningrad. He asked a group of professors there whether they had thought about what happens when man dies. After a few minutes discussion, one of the professors quietly went inside and came out with the book "Autobiography of a yogi."

He was surprised. In a country ruled by the materialistic philosophy of Marx and Lenin, here is an official of a government institute showing him Paramhansa ji's book "Please realize that the spirit of India is not alien to us", said professor "We accept the authenticity of everything recorded in this book, and we are trying to understand the state of super conscious this soul must have possessed while here in the body. Our research is focused on that.

V. R. Krishna Iyer wished there were scientific institutes in India that would have the courage openly to say, "We are doing research into the super consciousness of the paramhansa. But we do not yet have the courage.

education in human biomechanics and the study of human behavior under extreme situations is like being aware of how bud transforms into flower you cannot forcibly do it, it should be in accordance with the harmony of nature Students should be guided to introspect their vision to explore their full human potential by learning the art of relaxation by various aspects of yoga. The learning without competition adding the quality of feeling and ease, as equality and enjoyment of stillness in action are derived from a Sanskrit sloka "sthir sukham asanam" study pleasurable is the pose and the second part is "pyatam sathilyam anant smapatibhyam" meaning where effort ceases to exist or the state of effortless effort then you are in the way towards infinite. Movement should be natural tension free in a deep relaxed state. Exertion had to kept bare minimum because in yoga there no exertion it's not exercise, and acquirement of skill is based on the study of Indian Yogic philosophy, Slowly naturally developing into laws of interdisciplinary kinesiology, biomechanics, and psycho-physiology with easy yogic practices avoiding exertion understanding the philosophy because it's not callisthenic.

In Indian Martial Art, the main goal of a person is to avoid conflict by word of mouth or diffuse it by using nonviolent methods, avoid such places and situations at extreme situations just …….. Render the adversary harmless while minimizing losses for both self and foe. Students learn to be aware of self defense self understanding self exploration and be in the path of self realization work efficiently in any situation that requires defense, prevention of aggression, or conflict resolution. This is how the Indian Martial Artist takes an individual from action to liberation it's not to become fighters but to understand our tools to use at the right moment in self defense self understanding and self exploration.

Characteristics of Indian Martial Art

 Indian thought believes that god resides in every particle I have interacted with Dr Ram Bhosle a martial artist healer and the freedom fighter. He wanted to make a sitar an instrument to play music generally it has sixteen to seventeen stubs or gattas in between but he wanted to make thirty two, so he went to a tree and bowed prayed to tree. Which was situated at the river bank, the flow of continuous water was there underneath the tree. He requested to the tree that he wanted his wood for good reasons and then he made instrument out of that. Sir Jajdish Chandra basu worked to break the barrier between animate and inanimate by making his instrument kriskograph and proved that every particle has life we can understand Indian martial art by understanding the Indian healing or medicinal approach towards loving beings, the three approaches,Ayurvedic allopathic and homeopathic. The allopathic approach combats the symptom; the homeopathic approach amplifies and utilizes the symptom in the therapeutic process Ayurvedic goes to the root of the conflict because the rishis have understood that the five elements earth is enemy of water, water is enemy of fire, fire is enemy of air and space eats all. So they conclude three as the savior of the body mind quantum as in conjunction and they arewind bile and mucus. If these three are in harmony your system will be finely tuned. The yogic postures practiced have effects in whole endocrinal system to its brain centers if suppose someone is habitual bribe taker it's because some of his gland isn't working proper off course it has its past imprints in his consciousness due to the actions performed by him. Around the globe you can see the vast use of yoga and its relaxation methodology by some way or other, if you cannot do a normal exercise of stomach in an western exertion way you can practice same in a breakup yogic way all are using it except some like great grand master Bruce Lee may accept it and recommend Indian philosopher Jkrishnamurti for mental cultivation others start with their own names and country but Hindus are liberal to give out of love for humanity and by the way at death not a farthing can be carried away. What matters are your actions performed because they are carried away as imprints in your being. The Ayurvedic approach is seen in very few forms of martial art, for it orients not on conquering and controlling adversary, not on non-resistance and amplification but on going to the source of human nature's karmic juxtaposition as to why certain individual is like that because from one light all have evolved so who is bad or good under the roof of that one lord all are same.

In the entire globe land of ancient India is the only place where non violence had been practiced from thousands of years in the recent era Gandhi is the supreme example to conclude. Vajramukti is a non violent art uses body and its processes as means towards an end to know thyself and holistic healing. I am trying to describe or put my awareness of nonviolence, by quoting dialogue between Yulteshwar giri and Paramhansa Yogananda author of Autobiography of a Yogi.

Yuktesgwar ji was interpreting the ancient texts.Yoganandaji was also sitting there. A mosquito sat upon his thigh and was distracting his attention.Yogananda raised his hand, but at the same time he remembered Patanjalis sutra of nonviolence {ahimsa}.

"Why didn't you finish the job?"

said Yukteshwarji

"Master ! Do you advocate taking life?" replied Yoganandaji

"No, but in your mind you had already struck the death blow.

"I don't understand"

"By ahimsa Patanjali meant removal of the desire to kill"

This world is conveniently arranged for a literal practice of ahimsa. Man may be compelled to exterminate harmful creatures he is not under a similar compulsion to feel anger or animosity.

Patanjali yoga sutra 11...35 says.

"In the presence of a man
perfected in ahimsa {nonviolence}

Enmity does not arise."

This is the state true martial artist
should strive to be in it's the inner
state of developed mind

In evaluation as human we should
go away from war for higher
evolution

AWARENESS OF LITERATURE

The greatness whole ancient Indian literature was a ceaseless quest for the absolute. If you consider any subject Medical sciences, Mathematics, Astronomy and so on you will find there in essence it starts with that one reality. The whole Mahabharata is a Martial arts legend. But at every instance it takes you to higher awareness have you ever heard of at the midst of battlefield or fight someone is talking anout philosophy bhagvad gita is the written account of that. It makes you aware that we are not material beings but spiritual beings travelling in the material plane.

The best of the martial artist were masters in anatomy and physiology of the human body. They were also aware of metallurgy. They could make gold out of metals. The evidences can still be traced in the literature of Rama Krishna paramhansa the Guru of Swami Vivekananda.

Martial artists were helping poor people by curing with herbs and their talents of vibration therapy as medicine.

The different methods of self

defense which we call as "Martial arts" originated in India thousands of years ago. The Rishis mastered in marma sutras and other philosophical concepts of the ancient texts were teaching these arts to the warrior class of people. Apart from these, Yoga for its diaphragmatic breathing was an initial and a very important aspect of the art the concentration point was Manipura chakra. This chakra is the center of the prana (life force) within the body. It is responsible for distributing pranic energy throughout the entire body. One becomes powerful and energetic and tends to dominate situations by concentrating on this chakra.It is a symbol of agni(fire) and is very closely related to the sense of sight and movement of the feet, and is of very high importance for the Martial arts, no matter what style or country one belongs to. Although the Rishis were not stopping at this Chakra, because once you get some power and after demonstrating you get stuck with your ego and other factors, you cannot go to the higher levels. There are innumerable chakras in the body among them seven are in the texts as very important but there are more kept still in secret and practiced over in the Himalayan monasteries.One when muslim king Akbar was rulling he heard that someone at the cave in himalayas is holding tons of pappers which tells about every individual coming in this land of Hindus.Akbar went there was astonished to know everything about him including the terrain from which he comes was written in that.There was a man guarding these tons of pappers Akabar took these by force he distributed those among his hindu wifes and their relatives you can find these papaers scattered in different parts of the contry.

India is still a secret; full of mysteries. There are Rishis in the Himalayas still living from more than 4.000 years B.C. The description of one such person is given in a book Autobiography of a Yogi by Paramhansa Yogananda. His statue is carved and kept at California. He is still living at Himalayas. They stop their cells from disintegrating by the practices of higher Yogic methods."Martial arts" word has recently coined but in its purest form "Arts" were practiced much before that and same artists were also using it as healing art. "Martial" meaning is warlike representing planet Mars.

The monks were responsible for spreading these arts from India to other countries around the globe. Among them Bodhidharma is very prominent. These Monks were also in a position of breaking things without contact. They could just raise their hands and attack an opponent within the range of ten feet there are still Yogis living; who can do this.One such master named Prakasan is now using these powers for healing.master Bruce Lee was coming closer to this he wrote in his work from fist to elbow to shoulders much is lost but he left his body early.

In western countries remarkable works on alternative medicine was done by Sir Herbert Barker Master of Dr Ram Bhosle descendent of Chatrapati Shivaji Raja Bhosle.Another great work was by Wilhelm Reich (a member of Freud's circle) who first described character amour, the literal rigidification and distortion of the musculature expressing mental and emotional dysfunction. There

are many others working for
human betterment through
alternative means.

MARTIAL ARTS PRACTICED IN ANCIENT INDIA

Vajramushti

Mushti is a fist that is Indian fist fighting with a combination of Yogic methods, which was carried away by Monk Bodhidharma to China and was further named as Kung fu. Later on many local styles emerged, from that some retained the philosophical concept of the art and some were purely fighting art.

Varramanne

Philosophical concept of this art was same as Vajramushti. The difference was using of legs in a way of understanding sensitivity. These artists were using herbs as medicine.

Kalari

It is still practiced in southern part of India. In this a student starts learning with weapons including flexibility drills, and end up to an empty hand. Oils and herbs are also employed for giving more flexibility, toning of muscles and for curing of diseases.

Juha Chirakansha

It is another ancient traditional art. The movements were done in such a way as to integrate Mind, Body and Spirit for the development of an individual as a whole. It was also used as a form of self defense and medicine.

VAJRAMUKTI

Vajramukti is like taking a walk in the realms of the metaphysics of excellence. This encourages mental and physical progress of an individual soul. It teaches you to move from where you are. For instance an asthma patient cannot start from the same point as a conditioned wrestler would, nor can an obese person pick up at the same speed as that of the gymnast.

Vajramukti takes care of all, the gymnast, the athlete, the asthma patient and the obese person.

Needless to say there are therapeutic benefits as well, in the study of Vajramukti.

You will be surprised to know how this vajra word came to my mind. When I was studying in the primary school, there was a chapter in our text book about Maharishi Dadhichi. This Rishi had made his body very powerful by constantly meditating and yoga practices.

Vajra is the name of one of the major nadi which is directly connected with the genitourinary system and if you can consciously control it at wills, your body becomes very powerful.

At the time of the war between the gods & Devils, gods knew that Rishi Dadhichi s body can be transformed into a powerful weapon and used against demons. So they went to the Rishi and requested him for the betterment of mankind. Rishi sat on the padmasana, uttered OM and lift the body. Later on the weapon was made out of the body and was named as vajra and demons were destroyed.

When the body of an artist is like Vajra, he becomes physically excellent and this physical excellence can take him to metaphysical endeavors.

One has to be prepared to train his body in such a way that it could fulfill his desires for the achievement of the perfecthuman being, perfect in all respect and having control over his anatomy. Vajra is the weapon, and that's your body. What to do with the weapon is a thought left to your choice. Vajramukti makes you more aware about you and your body. But are ways and means to control and guide your entire thought culture, life style and the most important aspect- get to know how to think logic.

That is where the concept of "Mukti" or liberation comes in. Liberation is not only a mental process, but also a physical state of existence and a metaphysical quantum, which has to be understood. For when the consciousness of an individual practitioner is related to the consciousness of the eternal reality then the art of action becomes an artless art. This is what Vajramukti artists have to strive for, to become true artist or in the path of Tao or awakening. In awareness to deeper philosophical insight I am giving the question my father had asked me these talks will be on other book between me and my father as Svetakaetu Upanishad as my father wanted.

Shekhar Tell me about reincarnation and your masters way about renunciation, when I told you about mother's love. You told me about unearthly love, explain me about this love.

Pitaji (father)

Here is the dialogue from Hindu scriptures to explain reincarnation. Between king and the learnt man Bhanto Nagasana, does rebirth takes place without anything transmigrating or passing over?

Yes your majesty, a man were light a light from another light, pray, would the one light have passed over (transmigrated) to the other light?

No, verily Bhanto

In exactly the same way, Your Majesty does rebirth takes place without anything transmigrating

Give another illustration

Do you remember, Your Majesty, having learnt, when you were a boy, some verse or other from your professor of poetry?

Yes Bhanto

Pray, you're Majesty. Did the verse pass over (transmigrate) to you from your teacher?

No, verily, Bhanto

In exactly the same way, your Majesty does rebirth take place without anything transmigrating.

Bhanto Nagasena, said the king, what it is that is born into the next existence.

Your Majesty, said the elder. It is name and form that is born into the new Existence.

My master never advocates the path of renunciation he says you live in the world, perform all the worldly duties yet try to remain detached.

Within these karmic entanglements we have to find our way for knowing who we are.

My Guru says Mans life does not commence in the womb and never ends in the grave; it is the eternal quest or search for knowing the reality.

In one of those struggling years, I had no job whatever money was left. I utilized in two younger sisters classes. Also I utilized so much of my time to leave and take them.

This was due to karmic attachments. I had to perform. After this I had no money.

But my search for knowing myself was going on. The first lesson of yoga I had to give at lokhandwalla complex.

I asked panwalla. The man who sells Leaves used for chewing , how far is this address .Standing at Andheri railway station , he understood my position and wanted to give money to me which I lovingly refused .

I went walking till that address gave first lesson got money and started my days.

That time I remembered kuntiji's pandawas mother's statement that she wanted poverty because she will remember god, as god was there with her with all the problems she was facing. Many times I had not talked with you to make you understand this and then I wanted you to select wife for me and daughter in law for you so it gives peace to you.

I had to get this done thru same sisters who had poisoned our relationship.

Once when I was sailing on a ship named maharishi dayanand. There was a senior fitter he used to talk with his past births son.

At tea time he asked if I believed in life after death. I said yes more than you do also I believe in tramp souls or popularly known as ghosts. Tramp souls are the one who look for the bodies to make their vehicle. These souls are too much attached to the material world they cannot go to higher planes. There are souls of higher level who can come down from their planes and help the beings they are attached, Due to some karmic reasons; I believe his son was one among them.

He told me your people from hills are doing puja. I told him that usually happens at hills he said no but they are doing it oppositely or in a wrong way. He said that his son says they had been doing this from the time your parents had moved to Mumbai.

I phoned at Mumbai and

confirmed that yes they had phoned about that puja. This reminded me of Kashmiri girl who use to fall down standing straight as if she was empowered with some soul or controlled by some tramp souls .I had a strong feeling that this is due to the karmic entanglement of the past births. This kashmiri girl was cured later by one man who was curing peoples from such problems and this girl's schooling also had become better by that, but the man who cured her became sick and eventually died with his neck turning to one side. I believed that

that man had to take the karmas of the Kashmiri girl. Once at tea time on ship this senior fitter who talks with his past birth's son told me .Sir believe it or not your mother is feeding you and your father the tantric things which your sisters are getting. I got annoyed with him when he included my mother. But he said your sisters are giving to your mother by saying it's for the betterment of both of them. I was reluctant to fully believe these because I was following the path of yoga. I knew that these things exist, but I had strong faith on right path and action but I failed to understand the food which I had taken will definitely have certain chemical effects. I was facing many complications which I could fight with the help of yoga. But in spite of all this I was not against them believing this as a karmic conflict .I wanted to silently withdrew and within these problems I kept on my search for absolute truth.

Man's life is eternal quest or search for knowing the reality, unless he meets the perfect master who is lord himself, he only can take him to lord.

My master says resolving the conflict should be done to the

utmost level. We should do our best to avert any mishap in our families and should take care of our elders in every way.

In large Indian homes there is often a gate house- an independent accommodation built into the main courtyard entrance. Several generations would live together, & as the younger generation would take over the responsibilities of the family, the older generation would shift from the main house to the gate house. So one very cold winter's day, the grandfather of the family asked his grandson to fetch him a blanket.

The young boy went to his father. "It's very cold. "Said the boy to his father "And grandfather finds it chilly in the gatehouse. He wants a blanket to keep himself warm."

His father replied, "There is an old blanket in the stable, which the horses use. You can give it to him." The son fetched the blanket cut it into two pieces, gave half to the grandfather & brought the other half back."There was no need to cut it in two," said his father."I told you simply to give him the blanket "Well, "said his son."This half I have kept for you, for when you get old."

My guru clearly states by this anecdote. It is our responsibility to look after our elders, & we should take care of them in every way."

As we have talked earlier about parushrama as pitrabhakta devotee of father , you know I am also a pitrabhakta, but you believed mother as a greatest relation, both are valuable as karmic relationship but father is believed as the protector send by lord for us also I believed ultimate lord is father.

Pitaji if you read the book or works of Param sant Kabir says in "Anurag sagar" or "Ocean of love"

Brahma, Vishnu, Mahesh, sons of divine mother was very eager to meet their father Niranjan.

He had told divine mother no one can meet me. Brahma went for penance to meet his father but he couldn't meet. He lied to his mother about his meeting with his father, when divine mother meditated lord Niranjan refused about their meeting so Brahma was cursed by divine mother. Due to which he is not worshipped. Vishnu and Mahesh told the truth that they couldn't meet their father so they were blessed by divine mother.

This Anurag sagar means ocean of love. It is overflow of love from perfect Master Lord Kabir to his dear disciple Dharamdas.

These incidents given in anurag sagar were also narrated by Shri Hajari Prasad Dwivedi ji in his book Kabir

He writes that Sat purush Real God gave permission to his son Kal Niranjan to create shrusti or cosmos or universes. He calls him Dhurt Niranjan cunning one who did it wrongly. He was told to request and take the required material from "Kurmji"the second sabda or son of satpurush. Kal

Niranjan used his might and attacked kurmji, after destruction of kurmji's body the material came out was for creation

What I read in school about Lord Kabir and kept in my heart. About which I discussed with you pitaji, but you didn't understood. He described Guru in such a way only Param pita paramatma can be Guru. That is highest fatherly soul which is Real God as described by Hajari prasad dwivedi. It is the glory of the Guru "Sab sansar kagajkaru. Lekhani sab Vanrai, Sab samudra syahi karu, Guru gun likha na jaya".

If I make whole world as paper, make pen by utilizing whole of the forest, Make all seas as ink .I cannot write the quality of Guru. Lord Kabir himself was such a Guru and Dharamdas his chosen disciple.

Kabir for the normal people is an ordinary poet. But one who treads the path of knowing he knows and only he knows, if he never stops with simplicity of heart and soul, because his relationship with his lord is unique. It is like moths travelling towards light none of them knows about the other moth. They only know about light. Kabir as I read in school was found near the Lahartara Lake to Neeru and Neema named couple. They were Julahas considered as lower caste. They were earning their livelihood by weaving and making cloth at Banaras. At Banaras Ramanandji was a learned scholar, he was initiating by mantra only to Brahmins. Kabir made a hollow at his pathway to Holy River and slept there hidingly. Ramananda stepped at Kabir's body and uttered Ram, Ram, Ram. I got the initiation said Kabir and ran away; he started telling everyone Ramanandji initiated me. All

Brahmins went to Ramanandji how can you initiate a low caste to which Ramanandji said I haven't initiated him. Finally they assembled at court. Kabir was called, Ramanandji asked him. Kabir did I gave you mantra. Kabir said yes Guriji thrice; he got angry at a lie. Took out his (khadau) sandal and hit at Kabirs head. Kabir said sir now you have given your sandal of lotus feet's also. Ramanandji was shocked and understood the deservingness of kabir and said yes I have given you. From then they were to gether. Once while performing worship to the statue of lord. Kabir was sitting outside with a curtan between them. Ramanandji used to put curtain between them .Ramanandji was putting necklace on the statue which he was finding difficult. Kabir said while facing his back to him Guruji open the necklace and fix that, to which Ramanandji was shocked and said remove the curtain between us.

Pitaji Mother's love seemingly great it has higher value it has sacrificial feeling for the child .But it is not the real love, how can I make that statement? What is real? It is true, from where it comes? I will quote an incident from the time of king Janak to understand this. Janak ji used to wander at his palace at night time in disguise. In one house he saw from the window one couple was engaged in sex there was one lady also watching this she laughed at that, Janakji asked her why she did so. She said she will explain him after six years. After six years one female aged six came to his palace and asked to see him. After meeting she explained Janakji I am the same lady who laughed at the couple that night. That couple you watched were mother and son at their past births. They were repeatedly coming that way mother and son, husband and wife. I died that night fortunately due to some karma I remember past births that is why I laughed for they are into such entanglement and there is much to know. Pitaji Love as it was between you and I in search of infinite was of a higher quality. But Love, Love is beyond mind and matter and grows in the simplicity and purity of the heart.

That Love takes you to Satguru who is lord himself. Lord comes in the form of Satguru. Love should be like a moth going near the light not knowing about other moths. Radhasoami Masters say generally females go higher and faster in meditation. Because feeling of love is their abode. Same was confirmed by Paramhansa Yogananda author of Autobiography of a yogi. He said women's are dominated by feelings men's by reason. Both can grow by inculcating the quality of the other.

Kabir explains in love to Dhani Dharamdas O Dharamdas, understanding the reality. I am telling you about love. Those who meditate on Naam given by Perfect

Master in such a way that they forget everyone including their family, who do not have attachment of son and wife , and who understands this life as dream , are real lovers.

Brother in this world life is very short, and the world doesn't help at its end. In this world women is loved the most not even parents are loved so much. But the woman for whom one lays down his life doesn't help at the time of death. She weeps for her own self and at once goes to her parents place. Son kinsfolk and wealth are dreams, so my advice to you is to achieve Naam. Nothing goes with us in the end not even the body we love so much.

Kabir in the form of sat guru came in this physical material world. At the direction as ordained by Satpurush.

He was the third kala out of sixteen kalas or shabda,materializing from Satpurush or in simple words a third son of satpurush.

In the beginning Satpurush was in latent form as given in Anurag sagar. He had a desire and created souls. From his first shabda worlds and oceans were created, in which he dwelt. From his second shabda kurmaji was created. Kurmji caught Satpurush's feet and said he want to stay near him. Satpurush gave him the lokas to stay. From the third shabda, a son named Gyan was born also named as jogjit or Kabir. The fifth was Kal Niranjan,the creator of these material worlds. Sixth son was Sahaj.

The souls living in the meditation of Satpurush were very happy enjoying the nectar. In this way sixteen sons were born.

Beauty of these lokas or worlds cannot be described in languages, because it isbeyond conditioned world of mind and matter. The light of these worlds is not by sun or moon. To describe the beauty and love, I am quoting the incidence from ruhani diary of Radhasoami.

The Lord perfect Master
Shimla 31-10-1944

In bhajan I made some progress. I think. I had told you that I had penetrated the astral world and I had met your Radiant form. From there , after going through many beautiful places .I found the bell sound deepening into vast peals of bells and my vision growing clearer and brighter . I beheld such a brilliance as I could never have thought possible with this earthly mind. The inhabitants were luminous and bright and the dwelling of a design and grace that this earth will never know. I met and converse with the lord of that region. It was scarcely conversation as we know it. Words being almost unnecessary, a great deal by facial expression and gesture and a certain amount by pure perception from there I went into the Region of sunrise and sound deepened to a very deep resounding vibration. It required much concentration to pass through this stage. My artistic tendencies had to be purified. I am very fond of drawing and painting and the colors and forms and views were of a surpassing loveliness which held me down a long time.

I think, I must have explored this entire plane. Finally, I left it and lately more so at the Dera elsewhere. I have felt that vision i.e. earthly vision as such has been shed, feeling as we know it here has gone, and hearing is different. Contact with other souls [who are very bright indeed and very much a part of one, oneself] is by direct perception and above all I feel one with everything I meet [even here when I return to this body] out with you my beloved father, indeed am beginning to realize the meaning of that unearthly love which I have sought for so long. Very humbly I lay this little love at your feet. Several times I have come to the great darkness dear Master but I am still a coward. Please help me with strength. My concentration needs to be collected together very much more than I am doing here and I am weak as water. I have always been afraid of the dark and it will require some doing.

Pitaji it was this unearthly Love I was talking about, when I was under training with naval shipyard.This experience was from the highest form of meditation.

BRIEF LITERATURE OF OTHER ARTS

Other arts practiced around the

world were also having philosophical touch. Such as Zen therapy used by martial artist Tanyo roshi at Hawaii. My friend Michael Trembath practiced and learned under him. Later on when he came at Mumbai to learn from Dr Ram Bhosle student of Sir Herbert Barker, we became friends also I helped him with stories on Dr Ram Bhosle for writing the book. And spend lot of our time together at Shri Gagangiri Maharaj ashram.Gagangiri ji was a mystic and a spiritual healer. He was a living siddha an accomplished one. Scientists and Doctors used to visit him and we were interacting and exchanging our views. My Yoga teacher Alka tai was regularly practicing with Dr Ram Bhosle.I was going there and staying for hours just listening for maximum time and interacting at the end. Conclusion was live life logically to the fullest.

The contribution of western Masters like Ida Rolf is great in the field of alternative to medicine. Ida being a PhD in organic chemistry from Columbia University had practiced yoga asanas extensively, and also studied osteopathy and Homeopathy. Her method is to balance both sides of the body with each other and to align the major segments of the body with the gravitational field of the earth.

Aim of Vajramukti is based on these experiences. And that is to know what lies in our innermost selves through performing Action and increasing awareness. Vajrmukti offers you a higher path, enabling one to avoid conflict through the way of Dhyana (meditation).It developpranas flow throughout the body, teaches to control the movements mentally which results in physical fitness. It encourages discipline and nonviolence.

Vajramukti stands at the highest because of the addition of Yogic methods to the movement art of defense.Self defense, self understanding, and Self exploration go hand to hand in Vajramukti.

In Yoga all the postures are performed in a way that they become meditation. These asanas are not just the imitation of animal poses; they have slow effect on glandular system. They are so designed that every asana has an effect on specific chakras and the related endocrinal gland, by understanding which one can relate his physical movement to the cosmic movements. Many of the movement art were holistic and spiritualistic. Many were more on self defense. I will quote on some of them to understand the concept.

Jujutsu

The literal meaning of Jujutsu is gentle Art. There were more than 700 jujutsu styles practiced in Japan. The technique involves kicking, striking, kneeling, throwing, choking, joint locking, holding and use of certain weapons. The essence of jujutsu was the ability to move from one technique to another as quickly as required to control an attacker.

Dr Jigaro Kano studied many Jujitsu systems, among them the two schools are kito and Tenjin Shinyo School. He combined the best of them and coined the new school Kodokan Judo. Instead of Jujutsu he preferred a word

"Do" that is literally, 'Way'. There were many Jujutsu schools indulged in dangerous practices such as throwing and attacking by unfair means.Dr Jigaro Kano was much gentler and was welcomed by masses. After formation of

Kodakan judo many schools merged with Kodokan except Aikijutsu.

AIKIDO

It was founded by Master Morihei Ueshiba in Tokyo in 1942. The principle was, with the help of the correct technique and the flow of energy, gently control the strong, avoiding conflict.

HAKO-RYU JUJUTSU

It was founded on June 1, 1941 by ryuho okuyama. The most

important aspect of hakko ryu jujutsu is, emphasis on the natural way of twisting of the joints in a natural direction

It requires less strength and is difficult to resist physically. Hakko ryu techniques are based on the principles of koho shiatsu, the forms of Japanese finger pressure therapy created by Ryu ho Okuyama.

ARNIS

Also known as kali or escrima is a Martial art practiced in Philippines. The history of Martial Arts of one Philippines has got a strong impact of the Hindu Arts. Among all the invaders of the Philippines, the Hindu king shri vishayana was the one who helped to flourish their Arts, Literature and Martial Arts. He also brought with him an advanced civilization, Alphabets, use of weights and measures and the astronomical calendar.

Impact of the Hindus was such that till today as Hindus were using the Sanskrit word GURU for the Master, this term is still used in their Martial Art, but instead of GURU now it is GURO. "GU"RU" means" dispeller of darkness" "GU" stands for darkness "RU" stands for light.

The very important aspect of the Philippines art is, each student develops a style as per the suitability to his or her composure.

After the Spanish invaders, Philippines who were practicing this art were outlawed and hence they were practicing the art secretly.

BANDO

It is Burmese art of combat. Its origins are to be in India and Tibet. It includes, kicking, throwing, Striking, Grappling, Locking and using of weapons.

CAPOEIRA

Brazilian martial art, originated from folk dances of Negroes, traded slaves. Seeing the brutality of the traders, they developed the dance into a combative art. In this art many of the actions are performed from handstand position.

HWARANG DO

Meaning "The way of the flowering of man hood" one can imagine by name itself what the art could be. It is education in its real sense. As the name of the art, the art includes the entire essential requirement for the flowering of manhood. It is a original system of combat practiced in Korea. Healing was an important aspect of the art.

HAPKIDO

Hapkido is a combination of several martial arts, namely Hwarang do, Aikijutsu and Teakyon. Its philosophy is based on the water principle that is for gentle attack, counter powerfully and for strong, receive it gently.

IAIDO

It is a Japanese art of drawing the sword from its scabbard. For the Samurai it was the art of sword drawing called Iaijutsu but for the Shinto schools, it was spiritual, the way of the sword "IAIDO".

JEET KUNE DO

Jeet Kune Do was founded by Martial artist, Philosopher and Super star Bruce Lee. Jeet Kune Do meaning 'the way of intercepting fist'. This is not an organized form of martial art. It includes everything to serve its end. There are no set patterns and rules but there are some approaches towards understanding one's body and its tools.

Bruce Lee's highest expression towards his art can be understood by following a few lines from his book, 'Tao of jeet kune do'.

"By an error repeated throughout the ages, truth, becoming a law or a faith, places obstacles in the way of knowledge.

Method, which is in its very substance, ignorance, encloses truth within a vicious circle. We should break such a circle, not by seeking knowledge, but by discovering the cause of ignorance".

He had limited number of students because he believed in direct relationship between the Master and the student.

According to him to teach one to be skillful is easy but to teach him his own attitude is rather difficult, and this is not possible with large number of students. For Bruce Lee, Jeet kune do was, means towards self discovery.

KARATE DO

Meaning empty hand way. Karate-do name was given by Master Gichin Funakoshi. He changed the concept of TangJutsu to Karate do.

According to Funakoshi, body was the only weapon involved in karate do. Its philosophies were related to Buddhism.

KUNG FU

Meaning 'Skill'. Although with its background with Indian Monks and their philosophies, later on it had emerged in various different styles. Most of them were influenced by the theories of changes, acting upon the principles of Yin and

Yang, which in Hatha Yoga is considered as Ida and Pingla or sun and moon. The harmony between the two keeps the body from diseasing. Other major philosophies by which some styles have been influenced were Mahayana Buddhism and Taoism.

Special meditative techniques, including knowledge of the nature of five big elements (Panch maha bhutas) were also involved.

While practicing, KI was drawn from the base of the spine Coccyx and circulated throughout the body, passing between the kidneys, in the back of the head and finally down the front of the body. The idea was tap the energy at the Tan tien cavity also called as "Golden stove" and this pranic power was drawn from the Tan-tien to the palm of the hand.

WINCHUN KUNG FU

Most famous martial art, famous for its simultaneous attack and defense techniques "Chi sau" meaning sticky hand training, is a very important aspect of the art. If performed slowly if increases the sensitivity and the awareness of one's own and opponents movements and also strengthens the upper body. Trapping is a very peculiar art in this system and very effective for close range combats. It includes thrusting fingers that is finger strikes. It is believed that Wing Chun originated in the Honan province, at the Shaolin temple. Shaolin temple was also place for revolutionaries and secret societies. They were dedicated to finish the cruel dynasty. The then existing government had professional soldiers, highly skilled in martial arts and were putting a halt to the monks activities. So all the elders of the temple had a meeting in a hall and each one revealed his or her finest secret fighting techniques. The aim was to create a new art which would overcome all others and will be learned in a short time. The hall was named as wing Chun hall. After some time the temple was attacked by soldiers and many residents were killed in the attack.

A femalenun named Ng Mui was the sole survivor.Another belief is she developed the art after studying the discrepancies of other arts. She taught this art to Yip Man the master of Bruce Lee. While my study with other oriental arts I found this art more straight to the point has only one form known as little idea. Even with these the adept master Bruce Lee found himself trapped in classical mess so he came up with his art "Jeet kune do". Within the very small span of his life master Lee gave a lot to the world. His art is not just the fighting art it's the means towards self discovery for every individual. I started my journey deeper into metaphysics after reading his book "Tao of Jeet kune do".

JAPANESE EQUIVALENT, INDIAN LINGUISTIC &

THERAPEUTIC BENEFITS OF VAJRAMUKTI

The Japanese equivalent word for martial art is known as

"BUDO" which has got a very deep meaning, to know that one has to understand something about language. Language is based on signs and conventions. Chinese and Japanese languages are not designed as by western linguistics. If Chinese or Japanese wants to write a word for example 'Vessel', they will set up their sign and convention as per the vessel, closely related to the picture of the vessel. Therefore we see their language as a beautiful art work. The first character 'BU' in 'BUDO' is made up of two characters. The first character means 'to stop'. The second character is a symbol of spear. So it is 'to stop the spear' and 'DO' means the way for which the Chinese word is 'Tao'. So the meaning is' the way to stop the spear'. It is the way to cut down the disharmony, a way towards peace.

Something very interesting to mention here is about the Indian languages specifically Sanskrit and Hindi. These languages are not based as per any linguistic of the world. These languages are designed by exploring within the inner self. The masters explored the Yoga nadi, which are not the nerves, arteries and veins that are described by the Anatomist and Physiologists. These could be explored by psychoanalysts; they are working in that direction, Swami Rama at Pennsylvania had done extensive research helping scientists also. Body consists of many chakras. Each chakra is represented by a lotus. It has a particular number of petals with a sound emanating from that which Rishis had noted that in Sanskrit script. The number of petals in each chakra is determined by the number and position of the Yoga nadi around the chakra. The vibration is produced at each petal which is represented by the corresponding Sanskrit letter.

The related chakra and the fifty alphabets of Sanskrit are described further.

Mooladhara chakra:

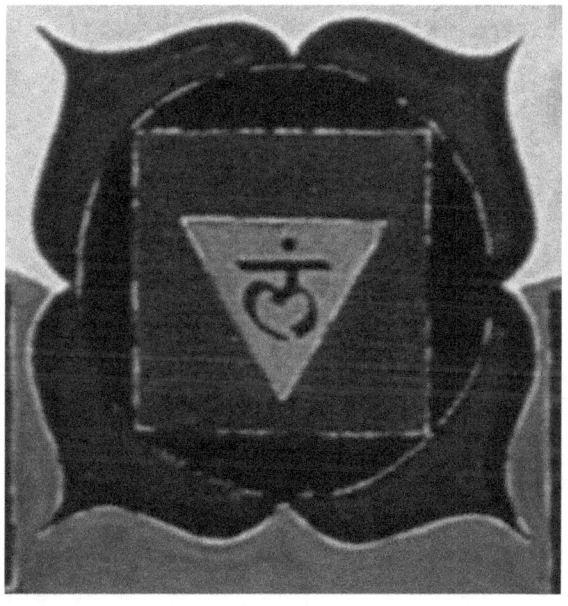

It is located at the base of the

spinal column. It is the lowest of the chakras. "Mool" means root. "Adhara" means support. It lies between the origin of the reproductory organ and the anus.

From "Mooladhara", chakra four important "nadis" or subtle channels emanate, which appear as the petal of lotus, which is symbolized by a deep red color. The subtle vibrations that are produced by each nadi are represented by the Sanskrit letters.

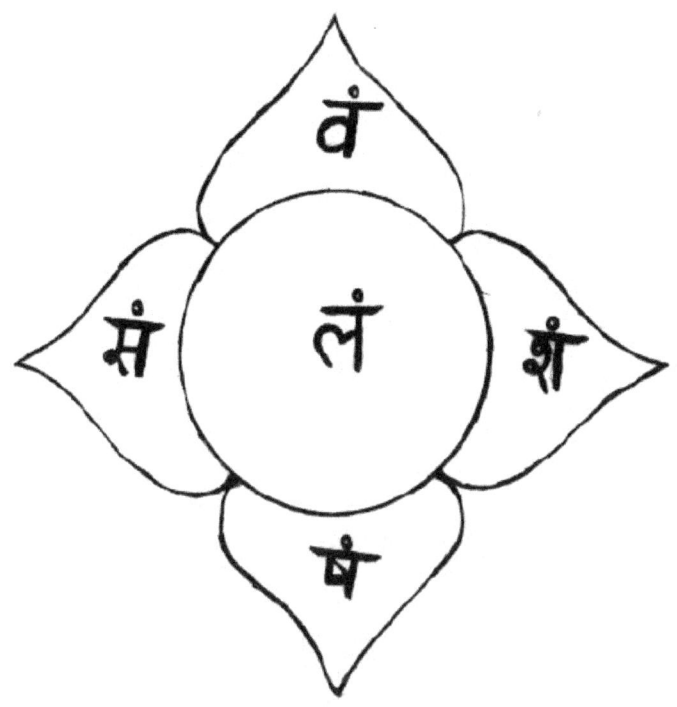

Here in this chakra "Kundalini" a serpent power lies dormant. It is believed that divine power lies here in a form of coiled serpent. The scriptures say one who penetrates this chakra conquers the "prithvi" tattva or earth element. He has no fear of death from earth.

Swadhisthana chakra:

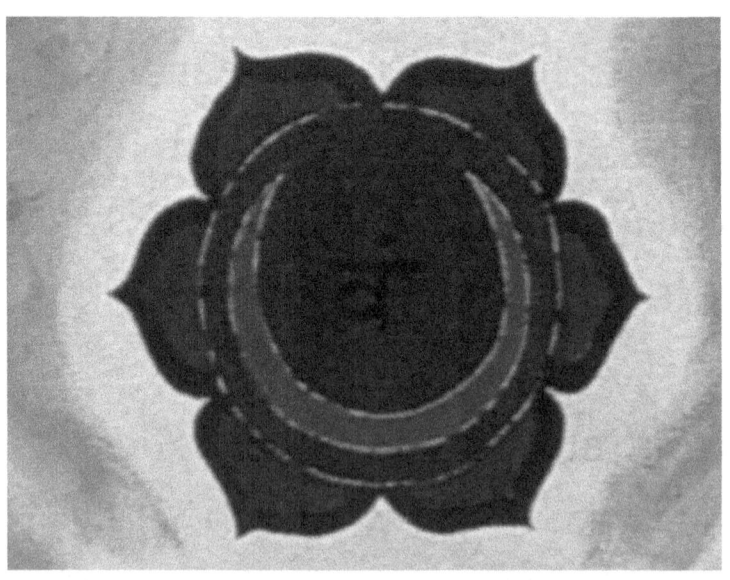

Swadhishthana chakra is above the mooladhara that is at the root of the reproductory organ. Swadishthana meaning one's own abode. The vibration produced by the nadi and the letters formed in each petal.

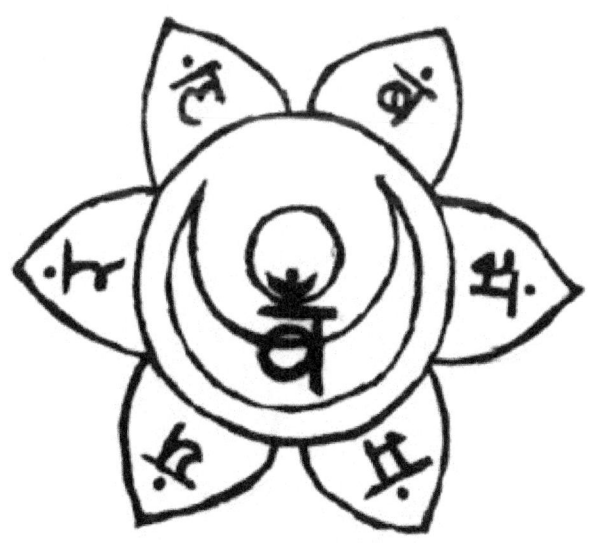

It is

associated with the organs of excretion and reproduction. He who concentrates on this chakra has control over water element.

Manipura chakra:

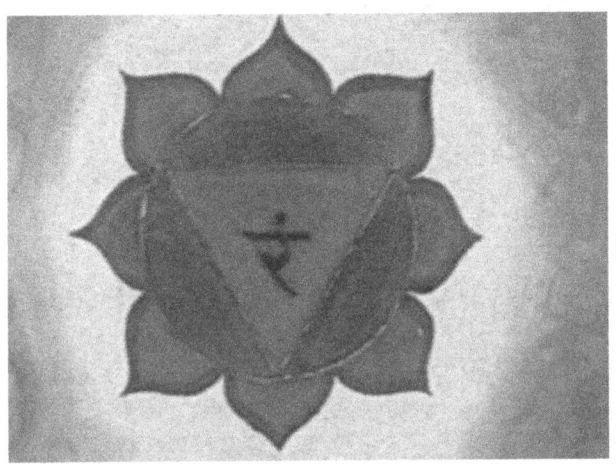

Manupura meaning, 'City of jewels' it is the third chakra from moolabandha. This chakra is a fire center. It is locatedat the nabhi sthana (Naval region).

The adrenal glands located above the kidneys are a gross

manifestation of Manipura. They secrete adrenaline into the blood stream during emergency situations. In effect, it speedup all the physiological processes, making the body ready for any intense activity, such as somebody all of a sudden attacking. From this chakra emanate ten yoga nadis which appear like the petals of lotus.

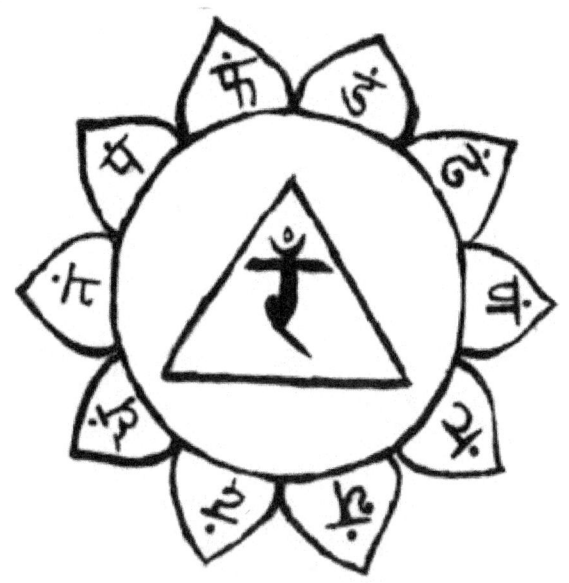

The vibrations produced are written and represented by the Sanskrit letters one who concentrates on this chakra can acquire hidden treasures and get control over fire element.

Anahata chakra:

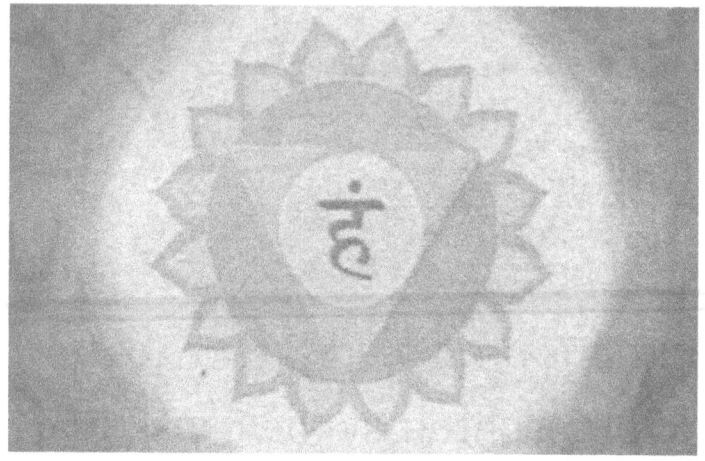

Anahata means sound produced without striking. All sounds are produced striking together of the objects. But Anahata is a soundless sound which is beyond material awareness, which is heard when you start exploring inside.

This chakra has control over heart. One who concentrates on this chakra gets control over the air element, (vayu tatva).

As per ancient text Gherand samhita he can fly in air, enter in another body. That is also known as parkayapravesh, it was demonstrated by Swami Rama's Guru. Given in the book living with Himalayan masters published from United States Pennsylvania. The sound produced and letters written are from twelve petalled

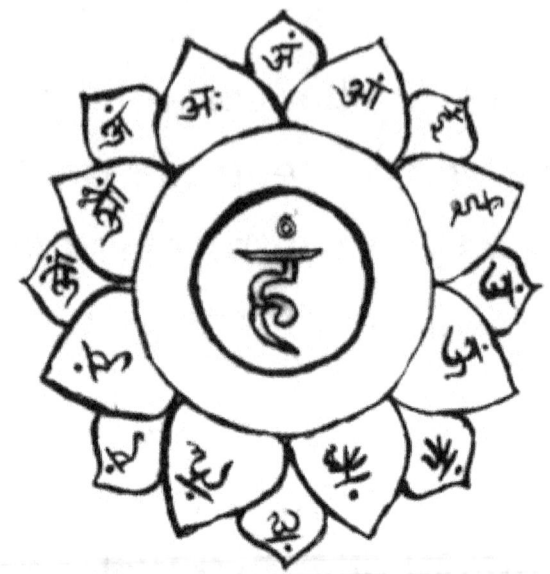

lotus.

Vishuddha chakra

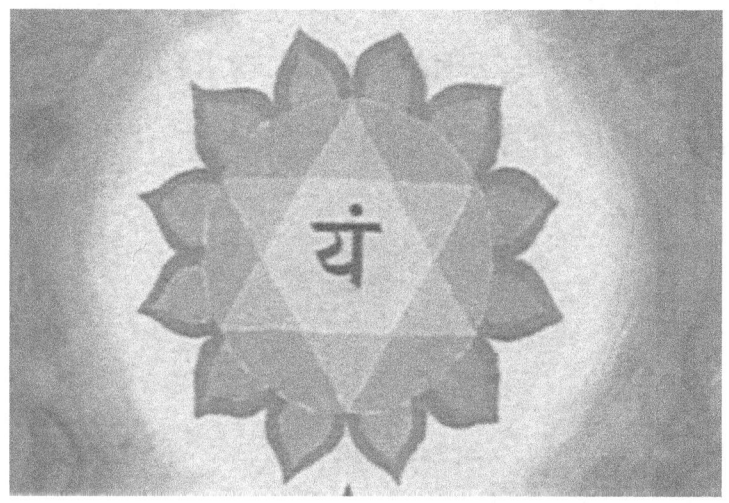

Vishuddha meaning purified.Vishuddha chakra is the center of purification process. It is situated at the base of the throat.

Sanskrit letter that emanate from the lotus is of sixteen petals so there are sixteen letters. One who concentrates on this chakra gets control over akasha tattva that is sky element or ether element.

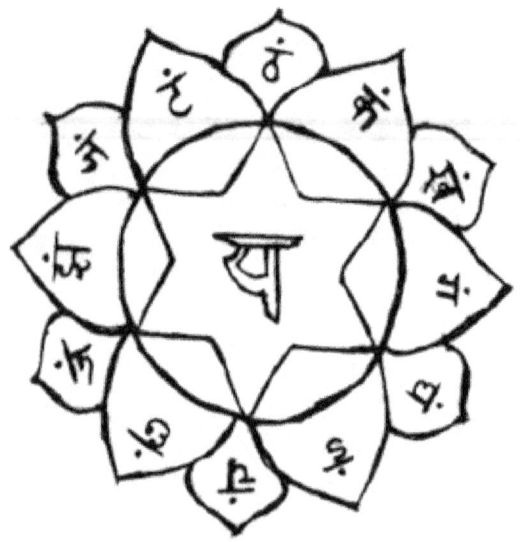

Scriptures say he will get full knowledge of Vedas and will know the past present and the future.

Ajna chakra

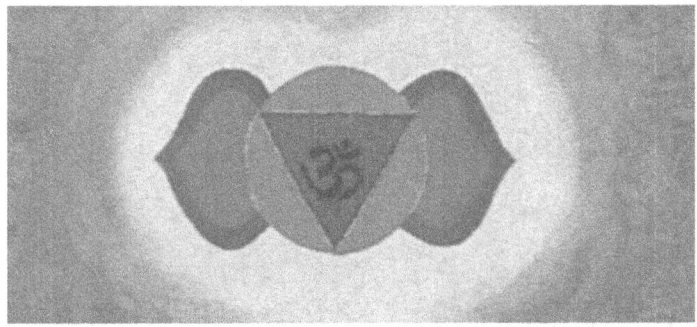

Ajna chakra is also known s the third eye or Shiva's eye Trikuti or triveni. Even Bible speaks about this chakra in Mathew 6.22. "When thine eye will be single, thine whole body will be full of light." This center is also known as bhrumadhya, the center between the hairlines above eyes.

In Bhagwad Gita it is deeply described in the 15th chapter 16th sloka. This is a point where kriya yogi meditates (Kriya yoga a higher Yogic sciences).

Ajna means permission. This is the center where eternal light is there and from here one is permitted to go to the higher state. The primal sound, the eternal word AUM is the central sound of this chakra. The lotus here is of two petals and the Sanskrit letters emanated are

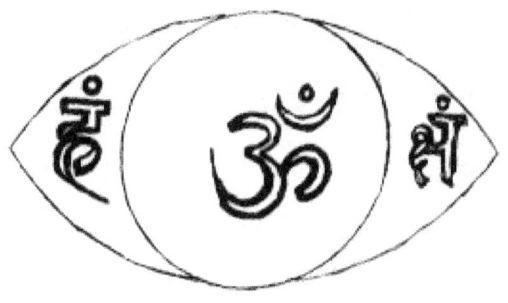

he who concentrates on this chakra destroys all the karma of the past lives as per the scriptures.

These nadi about which much has been said until now are subtle channels for the flowing of pranas currents. The human body is full of innumerable such nadi. If it is revealed to an individual, he will be witnessing his body as if he is looking at a vast universe.

The vibration and the sound produced are divided into four levels. They are paravani, pasyanti vani, Madhyama vani, and vaikhari vani. The primal sound is known as para vani.

Pashyanti is a state of sound which has color and form.Madhyama vani is a intermediate state and vaikhari is the grossest expression of sound which can be molded into any form of sign and convention, depending upon the environmental conditions and it becomes a language. Sound and light are the very important aspect to express the articulation of any art.

SEXUAL BENEFITS FROM VAJRAMUKTI

In the view of Ayurvedic masters, everything is a medicine

He may use sunlight, Mud, Herds or fresh air & Yogi will add pranayama in conjunction with them & if Tantrik awareness is added to it, this make an integral part of vajramukti & affects the cure. If we go deep further a thought is also a medicine. It consists of minute spandans (Vibrations) which has the power to heal or kill.

Ayurveda is composed of two terms, Ayus meaning life & Vedas meaning knowledge or science. Thus etymologically Ayurveda means life science or Biology. Various other aspects related to human life are included in ayurveda. It deals widely with the treatment of animals and plants. The very deep interrelation between yoga & Ayurveda is based on glandular functioning of the body. They can be of help to each other in such a way that any disease can be cured, without any surgery and side effects of the medicines. In ancient times there were many specialized subjects. Ayurveda provides rational means for the treatment of many internal diseases which are considered to be incurable in other systems of science.

As per yogic philosophy, the human body is composed of five big elements (Pancha mahabhuta). They are earth element (prithvi tattva), Air element (vaya tattva) ,water element (jal tattva), fire element (agni tattva),Sky or ether element (Akash tattva).All the particles in the universe is comprising of these five big elements.

The modern medicine may stimulate the nervous and glandular systems of the body, but the ultimate judgment is given by the Mind and it depends upon the capacity of the mind. The physical body consists of cells composed of protons, electrons, neutrons& so on in motion. These minute particles are the manifestation of thought. If we still move deeper inside, it is an idea which affects the thought process.

Therefore the Rishis had studied and divided the body into four parts, Sthula, shukshma. Karan, mahakaran that means sthula is gross and suksham meaning subtle body for subtle plane traversing karan and mahakaran are further subtle bodies. Partial tension is always there in the body. Even at the time of relaxation, mind is engaged in a thought and as a result some parts of muscles are tensed. Suppose an individual is talking to somebody. He won't be aware, unconsciously he might be tensing his right or left scapula, but if he tries to listen to his own talk and if he becomes the witness' of his body actions or body as a whole, he will notice, unknowingly he was tensing some part of his body which was not required. One has to remove all tension and send relaxed vibrations to the muscles and joints with the help of subtle yogic movements. This way we are doing the maintenance of the body.

Hatha yogis of ancient India discovered mudra and bandhas for rejuvenating glands to control and correct the over and under activity of the glands. One will get astonished by the deep knowledge of physiology an anatomy in subtlety of Rishis. If mangal granthi (Thymus gland) is not normal, the man can become thief a dacoit a murderer.If shivasati granthi (Pituitary gland) is abnormal, he may become a black marketer, habitual bribe taker etc. So enough is there in the body itself to cure its dis easing using medicine at extreme emergency to conclude Vajrmukti can reform human beings. As prana (vital Energy or ki) is very important for the practioner of Martial Arts, pranayama is to be understood. But before understanding pranayama, the incorrect chemicalization of the joints has to be corrected. In all our joints there is a stagnation of some air, the chemicalization of which can lead to many problems such as stiffness, Rheumatism and arthritis. Although in yoga there is no place for exercises because when exertion is involved, by exerting one cannot attain the state of 'effortless effort'. But to correct this stagnation of air some sukshama vyayamas (subtle exercises or movements) are done with awareness.

SUKSHMA VYAYAMA

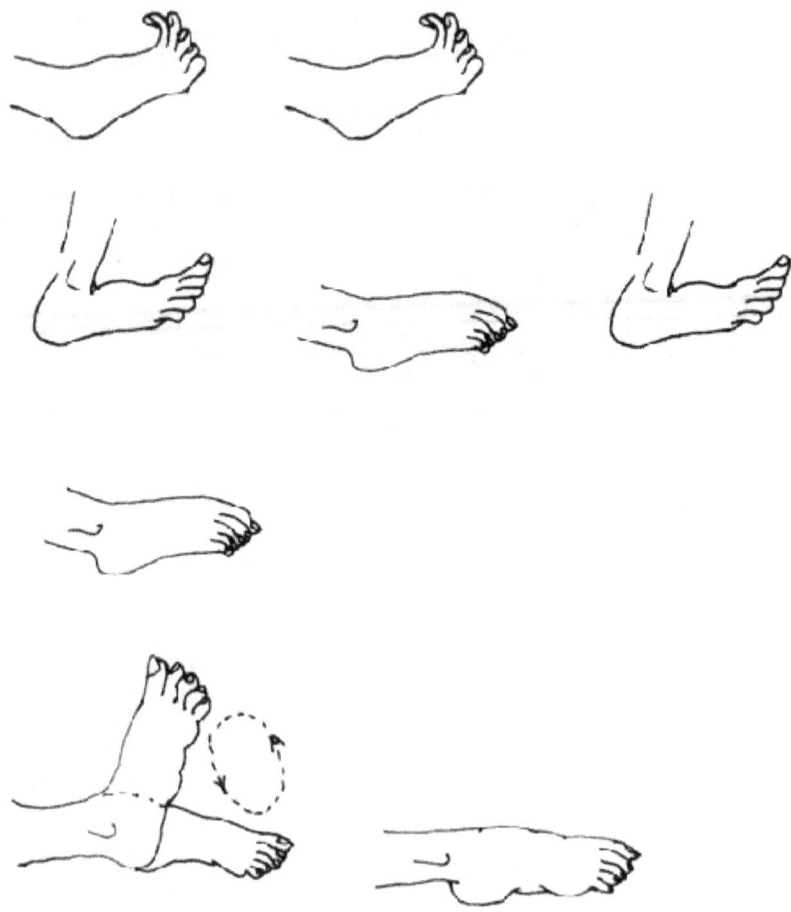

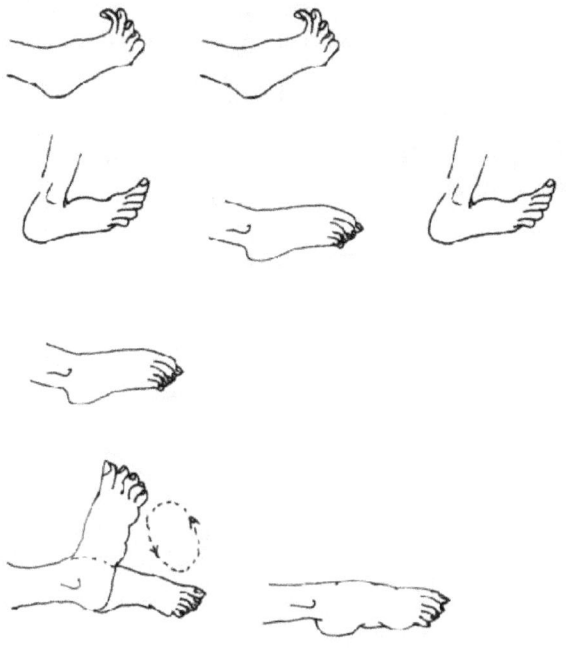

The illustration given above is toe bending. The idea is to put the total awareness on the foot. When you are using one foot, relax the other foot, concentrate on the big finger and then the smaller fingers successively and go on bending the fingers one by one, in the same way open them one by one. Circle the toe clockwise and anti clockwise simultaneously.

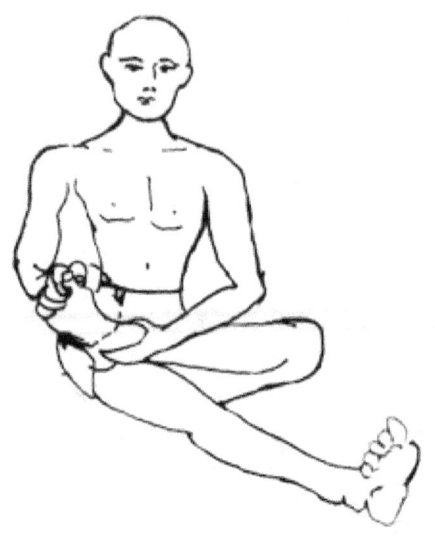

In the posture above, ankle rotation is been rotated. Sit on the buttocks, with both the legs outstretched. Bend one leg at the knee. Relax the other leg. Start rotating the ankle as in the posture, clockwise & anticlockwise simultaneously.

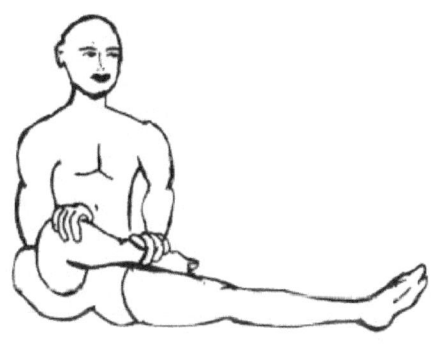

Sit on the buttocks. The legs outstretched, bend one leg at the knee. Place the feet on the other thigh. Try to touch the knee to the ground by slow & rhythmic jerks.

Do the same with the other leg.

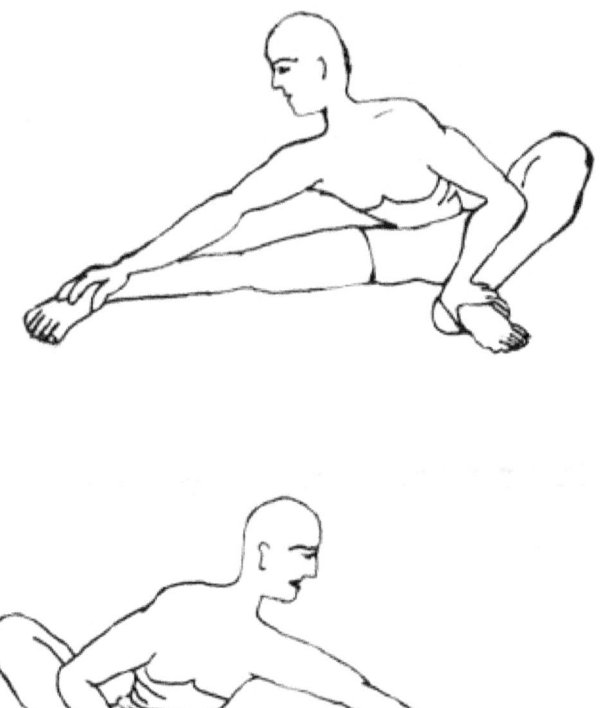

The postures above are deep knee bends. Stand with the legs apart. The distance between them may be 3 to 4 feet, hold both the feets with your palms, first sit on one side & slowly rise up & then sit on the other side.

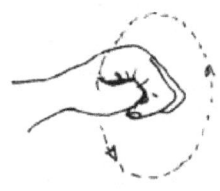

As per the illustration above, first clench the fist with the thumb inside. Stretch the full palm by opening the fingers forcefully.

As per illustration, now clench the fist with the thumb outside

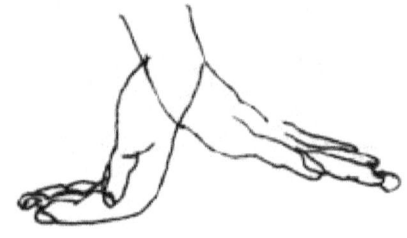

In this, bend the palm upward &
downward. Do the same keeping
the fingers bent. Clench the fist
and rotate the wrist clockwise and
then anticlockwise as illustrated
above.

Bring the forearms slowly towards
your shoulders and then, take
them away from the shoulders.
Circle your shoulders.

Move your neck foreword, backward and rotate it clockwise and anticlockwise.

Awareness of breath or simple Pranayama:

Pranayama is to learn control of prana or vital energy or ki

Lie down flat on the back, leaving the whole body as dead.

Put your mind on the naval. Place both the hands with interlocked fingers on the naval, start inhaling slowly and deeply through the nose. Imagine that the vital energy is entering through the medulla oblongata that is small brain or back of the head and imagine it is vibrating in all parts of the body including nerves, arteries, glands and the internal organs. While exhaling imagine all the toxins are being removed from the body. Inter locking the fingers, ensure that while breathing you are using abdomen first and then the thoracic region. So after filling the lungs to its fullest, while exhaling you can release your hands. This process will increase the amount of prana in your body.

CASE STUDY

This simple technique helped me when some kind of evil effect I was passing through. I found myself falling short of breath. Some people who do evil practices can send such vibes. I practiced the same simple technique and increased my awareness. I was cured. One businessman with the similar problem went to United States for getting cured. But none could understand his problem of breathless state.I worked with him for few sessions and he was cured.

PRANAYAMA

Prana is not just the air that we breathe. It is more subtle than the air. Although deep breathing exercises are beneficial they are not Pranayama. Pranayama works very subtly in subtle body and in turn affects the gross body. As per Yogic scriptures Prana in the body is divided into five sub pranas.

They are as follows....

PRANA: Controls respiratory system and speech organs, activates inhalation and exhalation.

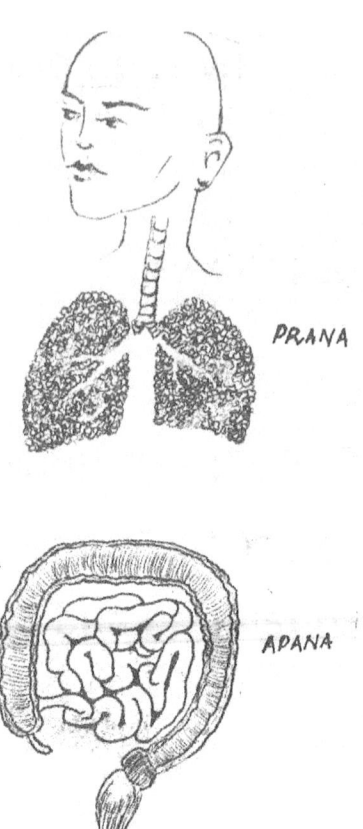

PRANA

APANA

190

APANA: Located below the naval region & it activates expulsions and excretions and helps eliminations.

SAMANA: Activates and controls the digestive system. It is concerned with the region between the heart and the naval & helps assimilation o nutrients.

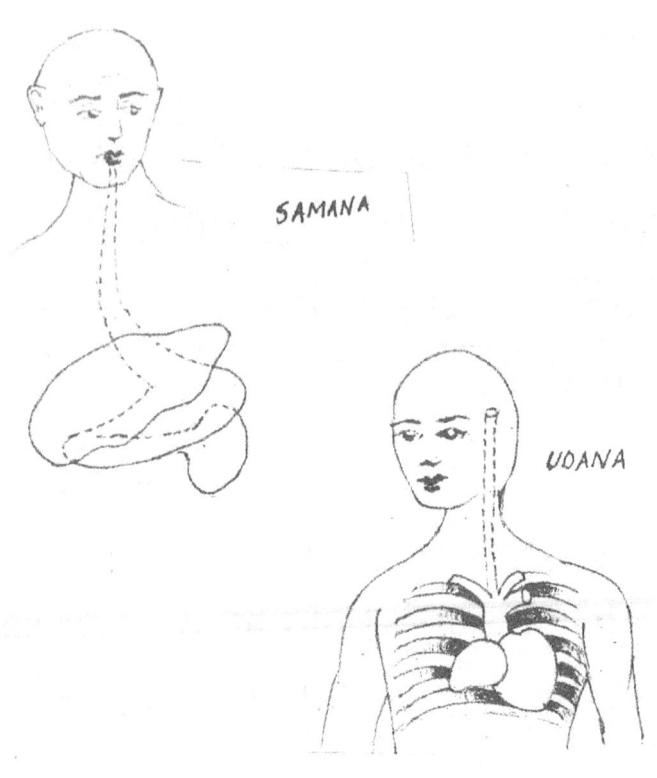

SAMANA

UDANA

UDANA: Dwells in the thoracic cavity and controls the intake of air and food, helps metabolism.

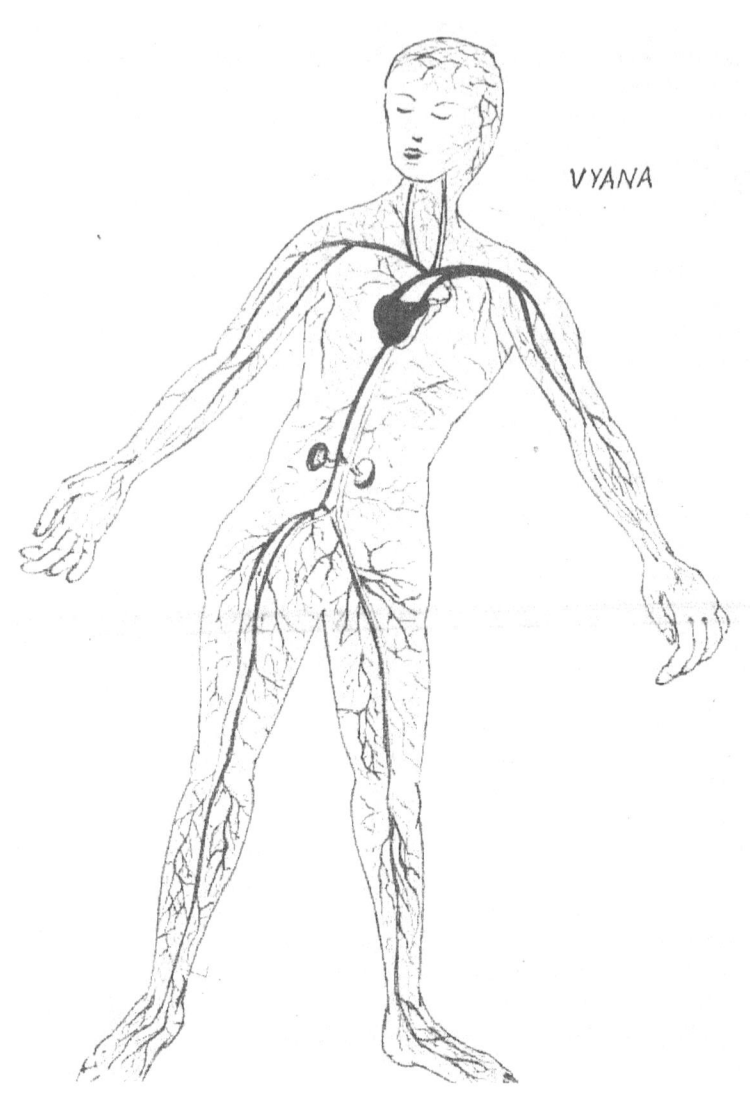

VYANA

Vyana controls circulation

Controls circulation

There are five sukshma (subtle) pranas as

Naga: It is responsible for relieving the abdominal pressure by belching.

Kurma: Controls movements of eyelids.

Krkara: Activates sneezing.

Devadatta: Avoids intake of extra oxygen when not required by causing a yawn.

Dhanamjaya: It remains in the body even after death.

Pranayama means to control the

prana vital energy, you will be surprised to know, when I was treating people suffering from various ailments, and many of them were not aware of the process that how their breathing is taking place! Either stomach protrudes first or the chest, while breathing. They were very much benefitted by making them aware and correcting them.

SEXUAL BENEFITS

"Sex" one of the most important psycho physiological requirement of human beings was never neglected in the Yogic philosophy. As yoga is the base of Vajramukti, it becomes an important integral part of it. As per the ancient texts and many seers, sex should be used only used for procreation and not otherwise. But it never happens, so therefore in texts of Hatha yoga pradeepika and Geranda samhita, they have mentioned that a person living a wayward life can also regain their energy by some mudras and bandha, accompanied by subsequent postures. Sex in itself is no sin, it is divine. We come out of the same sexual energy. The problem is, sex being a normal biological process, has turned out into a matter of prime importance. The reason is lack of proper education. When I say sex is divine I mean the same energy can be utilized for higher purpose, which is to reach to the super conscious state. The normal attraction between male and female is a biological process. Sex in not something sinful and to be ashamed, this feeling leads to concealment and hypocrisy. This attitude if goes unnoticed lacks the knowledge of sex for young ones, which is again not taught by guardians. The process of knowing each other goes in such a way that it makes the whole family a mess and an outsider exploits the situation an living becomes a misery later on in life. The whole living becomes hypocrisy. It is very strange, people hang on their houses. Love makes life worthwhile. Two kids, one male and one female kissing each other. But if you ask them, what is their idea about love? Is there any love among themselves or love is restricted to kids only or on show? They will be perplexed thinking that you have become a philosopher, because what they know is they do for the sake of doing, because other people do it. They don't have their own way of thinking and neither they are aware of the process as a whole. Living life logically at fullest is the way of being aware. If any thought is provoking. How is it coming? This is where the education comes into play and education is to unfold. It is not to make higher division clerks even if it is seemingly Information tech professional.

When one starts unfolding he is aware of his actions and then sex becomes secondary. Martial artists of the orient were at highest because they were trained to become a wholesome human being. They were embodiment of perfection and calmness at the time of conflict.

We come back to the understanding of sex. When I say sex is the psycho physiological requirement, it means it is physical and mental. It is a subject of behavioral science, it is psychological. But question is how much exploration of the mind has been done by human beings and above all, what mind is! Is mind brain or intellect? As per scriptures body is divided into five sheaths (koshas). The five sheaths are as follows: The grossest one which is the body is Annanmaya.Pranamaya is related with life substance, Manomaya, is a mental sheath, Vijnanamaya is related with knowledge or knowing, Anandamaya, related with bliss. Rishis believe that as the construction is in the individual's body, same is in the universe. According to them an individual is a small cosmos. What an individual knows is about the conscious mind, that too just a little. By the time he comes to an understanding of his mind, the process of thinking is already conditioned by whatever he has learnt. His unconscious mind is imprinted by a lot of past experiences, which controls his movements and he is confused. He plans something and something else happens. Now the important aspect is to be calm and aware. Ancient yogis have devised subtle mudras and bandha

By performing, even a single mudra can affect the related organ situated in the brain and as a result the instrument. Yogis say that any organ in the body is actually not the organ; it is the instrument of the organ which is situated in the "Bhramarandhara" or the equivalent word is Brain. Now suppose you have some mental problem, a yogi will give you a simple bandha a Jivha bandha (tongue lock), which is very important in kriya yoga (a higher yogic science). It is to touch your tongue to the upper palate of your mouth and stretch. You can see this in these two postures. You can sit in any pose back should be straight.

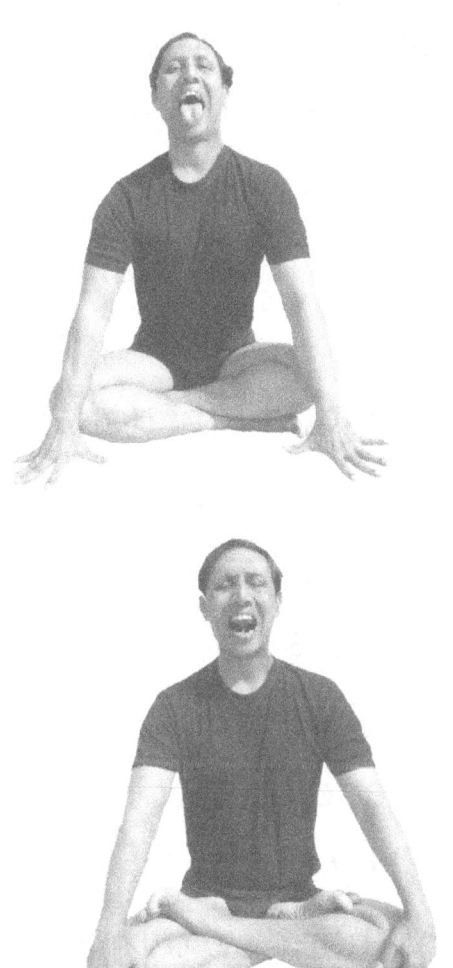

There won't be any harm by
performing it and if you are
interested, you can go for higher
meditative purpose also. This one

bandha has got a profound effect on vagus nerve, which is the highest autonomic nerve and it sends fibres to many glands and organs. The autonomic nervous system is divided fubctionally into two parts, Sympathetic & Parasympathetic system. Sympathetic system lies in front of the vertebral column and is associated and connected with the spinal cord by the nerve fibres. The Parasympathetic system is divided into two parts composed of cranial and sacral autonomic nerves.

These sympathetic and parasympathetic cords constitute

the Autonomic system which supplies nerves to the involuntary organs such as heart, lungs, intestines, kidnes, liver etc and controls them. The vagus nerve is the tenth cranial nerve and is associated with the medulla oblongata.Coming back to sex, for some people sex is ending point of love, for some love is divine and some doesn't know anything, they are performing due to biological need. Now the question is what this Love is, one can write a thousand page book on it, but still it is difficult to define love, because is to give unconditionally, without any condition. You will rarely find such a person who can give without any condition and if you find you are fortunate, because that person will be perfect

And as I have described earlier, for some people love is divine, now the word God (Bhagwan) arrives here. Let me explain you wahat this very widely used word Bhagwan is.Bhag is the Sanskrit word which means yoni or vagina & wan is the one who passes through.Bhagwan means, the one who passes through the vagina. But this is not a vagina of a female. This is the name given because it gives birth to a new human. The one who passes through the place between the eyebroughs.Now his whole body is full of light and he is the new one or awakened one. I read the translation of Gita by many authors, but was not satisfied, about the explanation of Karma and Kutashta, which only Lahiri mahasaya the master of master of paramahansa Yogananda author of Autobiography of a Yogi, has described in his works. Karma which can give you liberation is not by doing any work, because whatever you do, you will have both types of thinking, either good or bad and how can such karma give you liberation. For liberation is beyond duality. Therefore, the actual karma starts at the state of doing nothing that happens when your body is in the state of doing nothing, no thinking no reflecting, that happens when you enter inside yourself, then the actual karma starts. Scriptures say that one who passes the center between the eyebroughs becomes bhagwan, becomes one with the eternal consciousness. All the deities the lords of other chakras bestow blessings on him. When you take all this into considerations, love is for the eternal. One doesn't love for the lover, he loves for the self. But the self is to be sought Upanishads says. "When one sees the beauty, the eyes are trying to hold the beauty and in the process of holding at the beautiful object, the reality is moved from that". So love is for eternal, karma is for that eternal. Sun comes in praising of that one lord, so the moon, whole cosmos is singing in praisal of that one lord, then sex becomes secondary, but still very important because the same sexual energy can take you to the highest endeavors. Some mudras, bandha and asanas are described with illustrations and postures for sexual benefits.

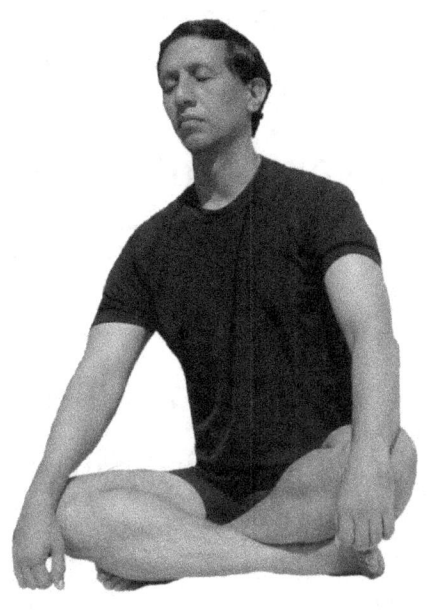

Sit in a folded leg posture or lie down. With a slow inhalation draw upthe sex anal nerves. Initially all three penis anus and the middle portion between the two has to be contracted. As gradually you are aware of the muscles you can segregate them.If you contract the penis or you pull the sex nerves by which you can lift it up it is known as vajroli mudra.and contracting and relaxing them is beneficial and improves the sexual controlling power.If you contract and relax the anus it is know as ashwini mudra it is prevential in many diseaseas such as piles.The third one is very important that is the portion between testes and anus known as moolabandha.

Same applies for females also the part from which they urinate the contraction and relaxation of which is known as vajroli mudra. The middle portion between the two is moola bandha the anus contraction is ashwini mudra. You can do forty contraction and relaxation. If you practice all these together it is known as shaktichalini mudra. When you strain the nerves start it for three seconds and gradually increase it.

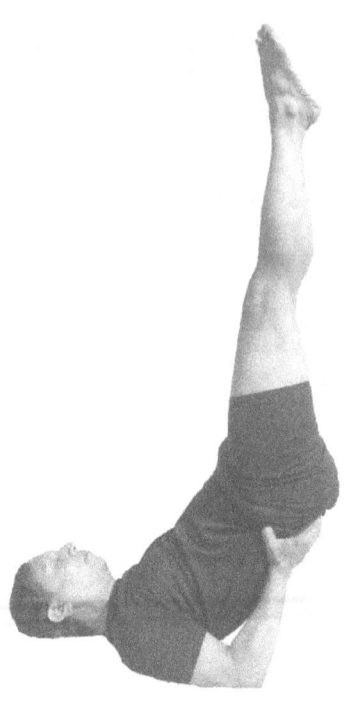

VIPARITAKARNI

The above postures is called as viparitakarni or reverse doing in english .Lie flat on the floor, bend the knees & move them towards the stomach. Raise the hips and legs. Support the hips with palms. The back is maintained at about fourty five degree angle with the floor. The throat is not blocked, hence flow of blood is allowed to the brain. This pose brings control over anal sphincters.

Improvement in sexual function of the body takes place prevents hernia. It encourages the function of the valves and the veins, hence preventing varicose veins. Gives tone to the abdominal muscles and keeps the uterus in normal state.

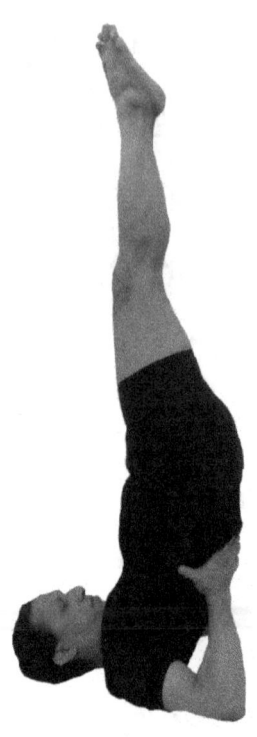

SARVANGASANA

The above posture works for all parts of the body.Named

In Sanskrit as 'Sarvangasana' or you may call shoulder stand.

Lay down flat on the floor.bend the

knees. Move them towards stomach, raise the hips and legs. Support the back with the palms.Bending the arms at the elbows, until the chest touches the skin. This pose drains the fluids from feet and lower pelvis, and the 'chin lock' the Sanskrit name 'Jalandhara bandha' prevents these wastes from flooding the brain before they are taken up by the circulatory system and is eliminated thereafter. The head stand 'Shirshasana' should be done after this in order to get a full supply of fresh, rich blood, flowing from the heart to the brain.

BENEFITS OF MOVEMENT ART

Movement art or moving meditation was emerged by the Masters of the orient due to long hours of sitting meditation. where you recharge your cells these movements are given in my channel playlist teaching martial arts please see https://youtu.be/yN79YV0dCMY

https://youtu.be/KE_Lsgog9ng

Origin of moving meditation can be explained as 'from formlessness to form'. As I have already mentioned that manipura chakra is associated with the sense of sight and movement. Ancient monks used to walk in such a way that they were becoming aware of the every instant of the movements of their feet's.By this slow walking and turning and putting ones awareness at the naval center, one can become totally aware of his body processes and surroundings, finally exploring the inner secrets. By making

Use of the form which is the body, they used to go towards formlessness.Kata in martial arts and dances done to express an inner state and to grow logically like Martha graham,

Isodora Duncan La meri, Balerina etc fall into this state. By practicing these in conjunction with controlled breathing it serves the purpose of keeping good health and self defense and self exploration.Monks like Bodhidharma used to sit still for more than nineteen hours requires his body to move slowly in fact with their awareness they create the movements for expressing their self as an artist.I am givng the poses below for rejuvenation or energisesations of cells.

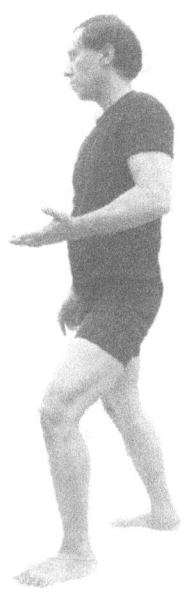

In this pose forearm and calf muscles of left side are contracted while doing so other muscles remain relaxed. While releasing visualize energy is coming from back of head through center between eyebrows to forearm and calf muscles and recharging the cells. In the

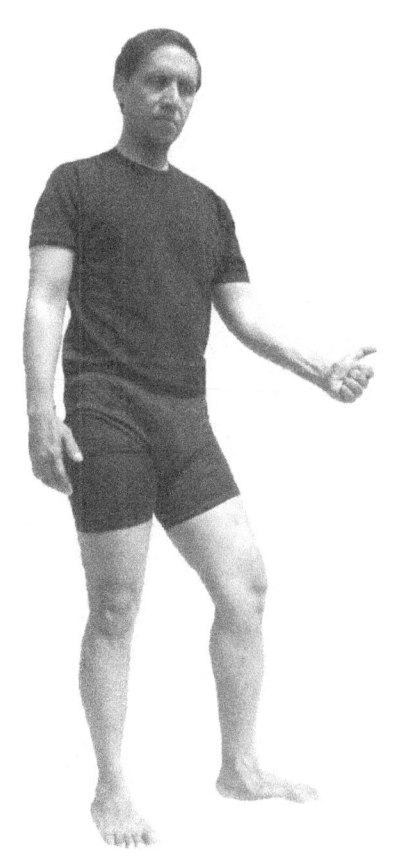

Second pose the upper arm and thigh muscles are contracted in the same manner.

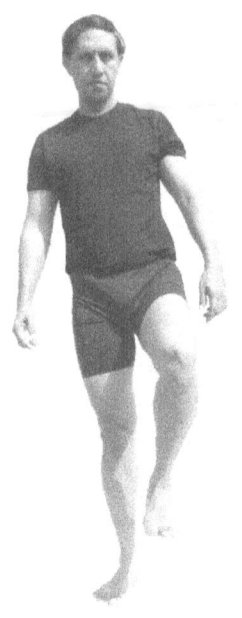

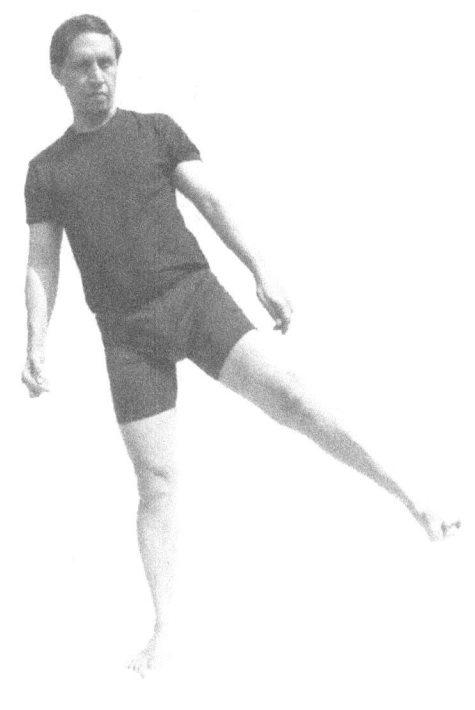

This is another pose for cell recharging .Fold your knee upward & kick sideways slowly contracting the muscles of the leg while concentrating at eye center or between the eye brows. After contracting release the muscles

feel the vibration & energy
pulsating as tingling sensations.

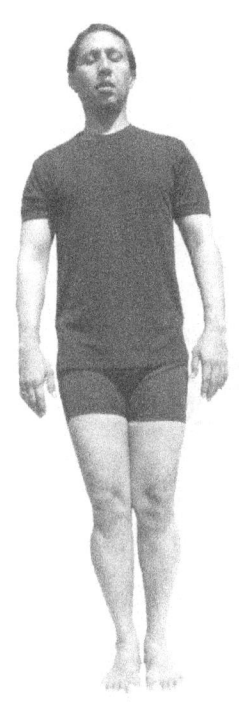

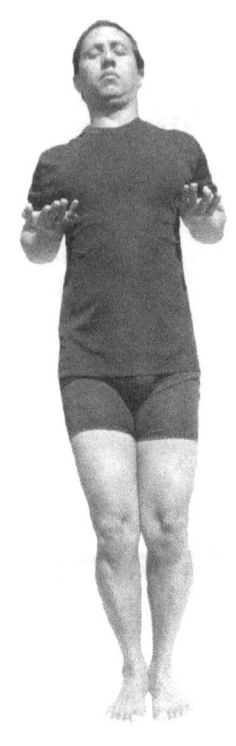

In these two poses first
exhale through the mouth then
inhale and start contracting the
muscles upward from feet's calves'
thighs buttocks lower and upper
abdomen take the palms at the

sides facing upward. Go on contracting shoulders neck and facial muscles till the scalp area keep it for twenty seconds then exhale releasing the muscles in reverse order as in the first pose. Feel that all body partsare recharged.

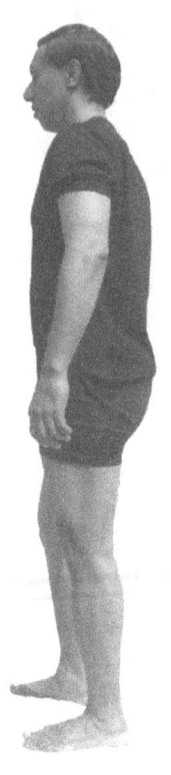

In the above pose put your body weight on left leg concentrating on your left buttock and chest muscles sothat you can contract left side buttock and chest muscles.Perform same way on the right side. While releasing the pose feel that the energy is coming from back of the head through the place between the eyebroughs and pulsating at the part which you had relaxed.

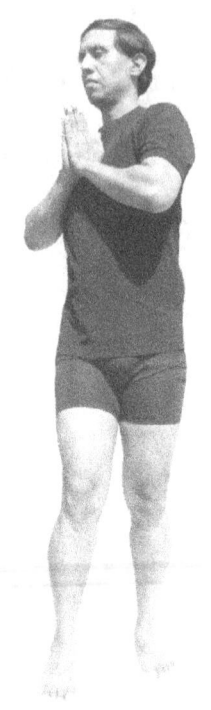

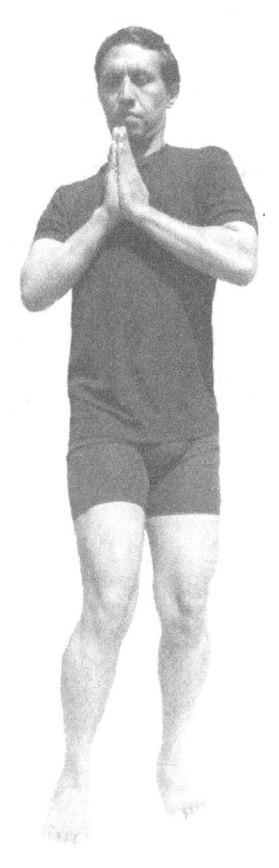

These two poses are kind of spinal adjustment. First rotate or move the upper portion that is shoulders to one side then move lower portion that is hips to other side.Once you understand this, move both to gether.This will remove any minor maladjustment in the spine.Virabhadrasana is another pose to correct the spinal maladjustment.

VIRABHADRASANA

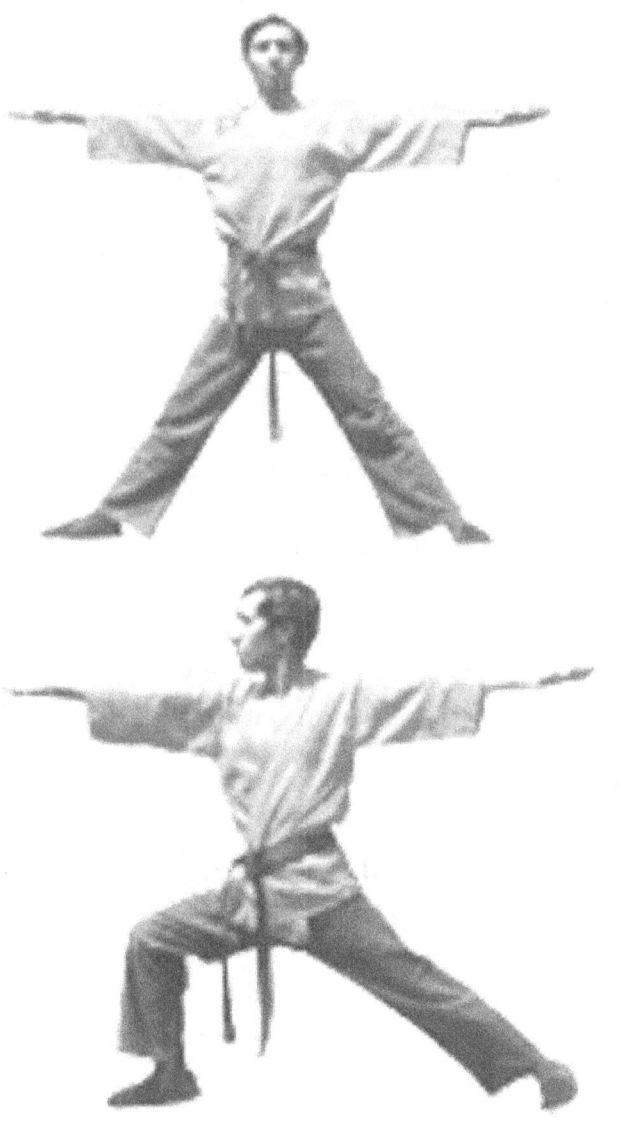

These two poses are known as

virabhadrasana named after a martial hero virabhadra.These are also helpful in spinal maladjustment spread your legs and hands sideways.Palms facing downwards stretched hands as if they are pulled.Turn face to one side front foot straight back foot turned inward,bend front knee shin

Perpendicular to ground stays in pose for short time or depending upon your enduring capacity.

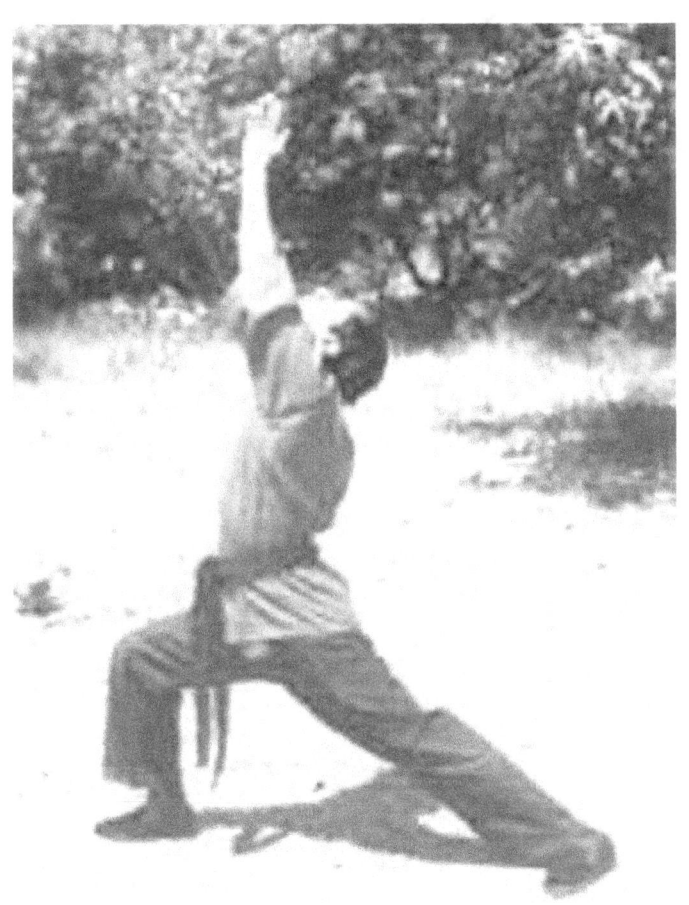

This is the third pose of the movement series.I had not cropped this pose so it looks different because here you twist your torso or upper body or hips touch your palms together tilt the head this gives the intense stretch to spine and hip muscles it also helps in removing minor tilt of the posture. These virabhadrasanas and moving meditation can be done after long hours of sitting meditation.

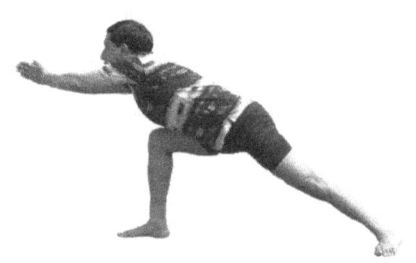

Place body weight on front leg by bending forward for preparing the easy lift of back foot straight at

knee

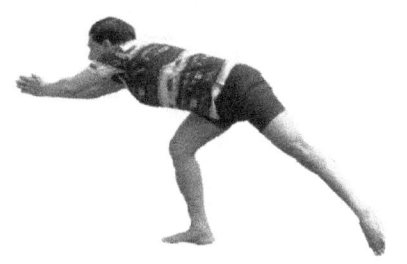

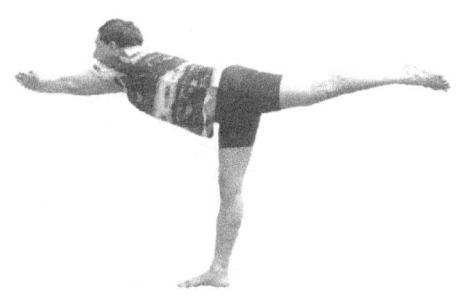

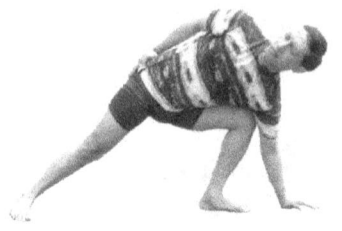

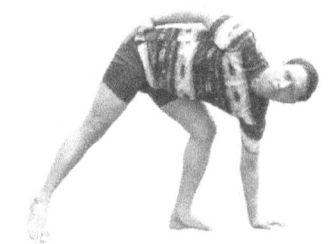

This is for side stretch. Place the palm on the floor while standing in virabhadrasana pose slowly raises the leg straitening the knees.

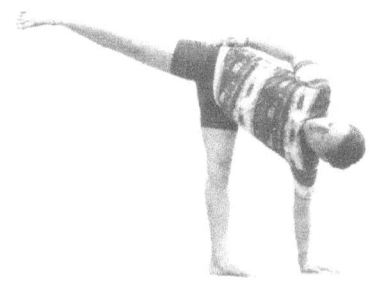

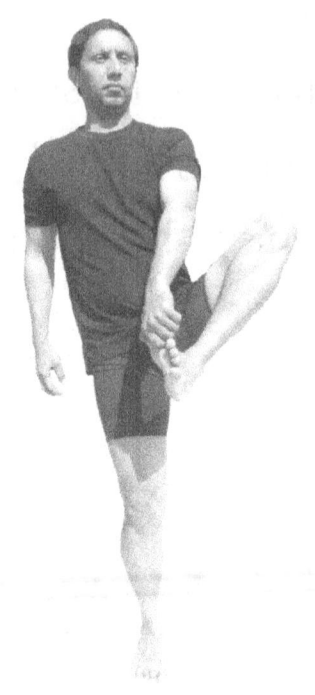

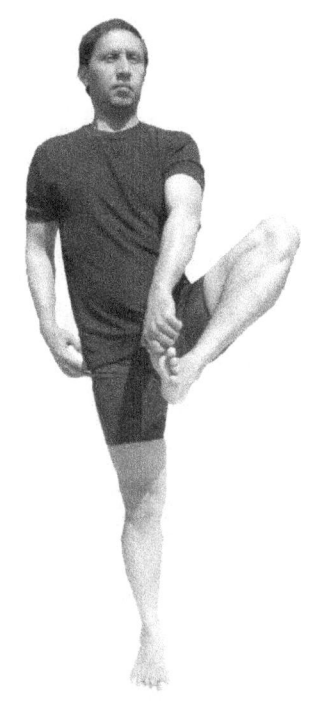

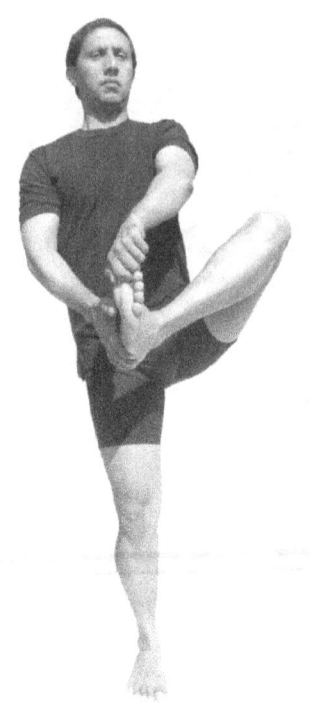

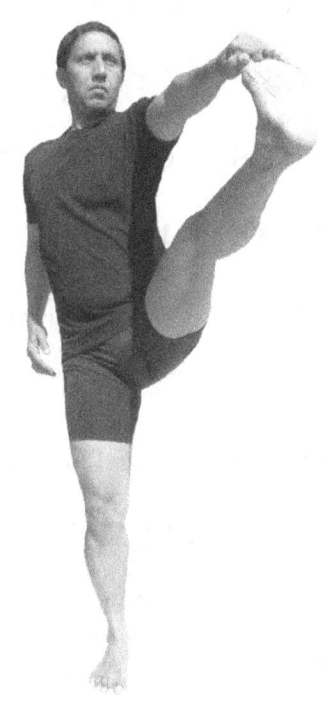

These four poses above are for increasing the sense of balance and stretching. Practice with both the legs.These all balancing stances or what I call is veerabhadras are important for moving meditation

Moving meditation should be done

after long hours of sitting meditation.I am explaining her how veerabhadras are moved and body is carried from one part of space to another.In veerabhadras the more weight of the body is on the front leg. This is just the little idea one can shift weight as per his requirement. You can put more weight on back leg and create your own moves. These movements are known as vajras they are nonviolent moves can be used for self defense, its main purpose is in aid to meditation. These are means towards end and not end. These should not become a conditioning.

Master Bruce lee said is style important or individual. Both has their value but individual is more important. The system which is moving towards deconditioning is more important.

Here in these postures moving meditation is started with vajrasana or kneeling posture. Let me explain how to sit in this posture known as vajrasana. Sit while your legs are extended in front of you. Shift your weight on one buttock and bend the other knee. Take the feet under your buttock keeping the heel turned outside so that you can keep you buttocks. Now bend the other leg in the same manner. See the pose.

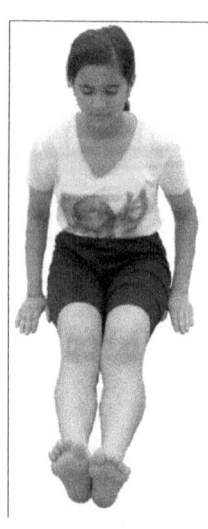

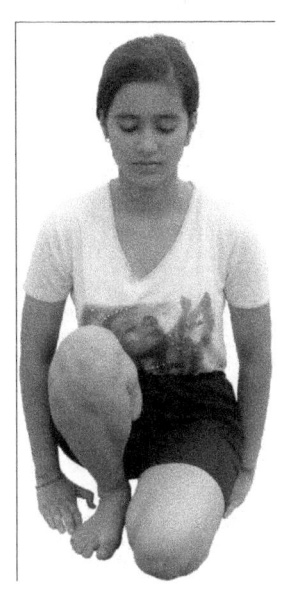

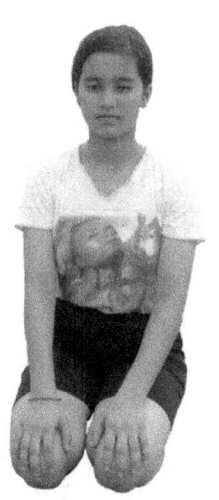

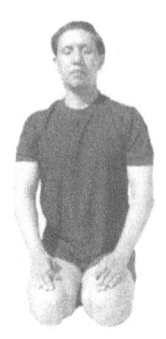

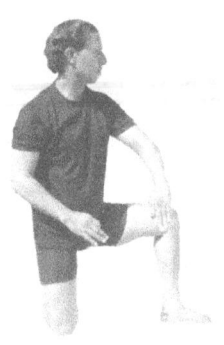

In this

peculiar mudra, the index finger is
making a right angle while
touching the thumb is known as
dhyan mudra.

Touch the thumb with the index finger, these mudras can be performed in any easy postures.

Benefits: It is the most important mudra used for meditation, helps in increasing brain power, prevents mental disorders, mental tensions. This was taught to me by a yogi Swami Chakrajit. He was initiated in the Himalayas. Swamiji was drawn by an inner urge to go towards the Himalayas. One fine day he set on his eternal journey, he never knew what way he was going, whether he had any money etc with him. He straight away went to the railway station. While entering the platform, a ticket collector stopped him demanding to show the ticket. Somebody showed his ticket and took him by his hand and made him sit in the train, in the upper class. He did not recollect as to how longhe travelled. Somebody woke him up at the kathgodam foothill of the Himalayas kumaon Range terminus of the East Indian Railway and took him to the bus stop. He knew not the destination of the bus but he was made to sit there and the ticket was handed over to him for the journey where he was destined to go. A six year old boy come up to him and took him to a place from where some people were about to leave for Kailas & Mansarovar. He could recollect that the place from where he started was Almora. He follows the group for quite a long time, mostly without any food. Other people used to ask him as to why he was in such a state. They were not convinced even after an honest reply to them that he reached there with a definite purpose to acquire some spiritual gain. When

Lake Mansarovar came, he was overjoyed and told the people around him that he had found out the place for whichhe was destined. He made his way alone through ups and downs, till he reached the deep Himalayas, where he started his practices of yoga. He knew for how long he was there. When he experienced the snow fall, he could recollect that he was completely drowned in the snow & slowly became unconscious. Then he found himself in a very big cave. He made it sure that he was not dreaming. He walked a while up and down the cave and then suddenly got startled and stood gazing, for what he saw was a sage sitting before him is a meditative pose. He could very well make out that his body was extraordinary. He was the most beautiful personality he had ever seen, about whom he very less describes. But his very personal students claim that he was sage vyasa. While gazing the sage he had experienced that he was completely lost and the sage had overpowered him. His body and mind started practicing systems of yoga. In practicing his retention of breath had increased to a very high extent to get all the extra sensory powers and experience enlightenment. He stayed there for six months after that he received an order from his Guru that he has to go back to the world of man. Recently at his residence at Pune he called his family members and left his body. He was very simple and humble people staying there hardly knew about his achievement.

Meditate on vajrasana index finger touching the thumb. Slowly rise while inhaling and attain veerabhadrasana on either side turn your wrist inwards. While doing this feel the sensation as if energy is coming through medulla oblongata or small brain and getting distributed through center between eyebrows.Bend your wrists inward feel the energy flowing as vibrating sensations.

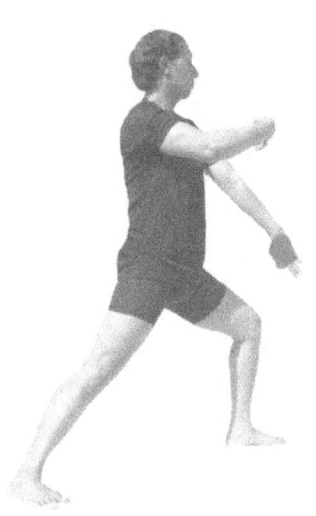

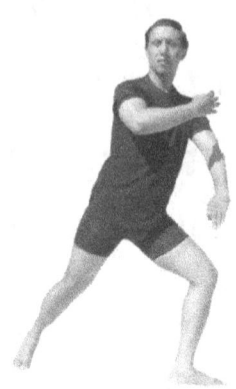

Make an arc with back leg and turn exhaling

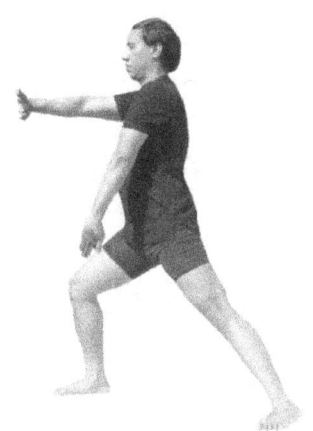

Co mplete the exhalation by feeling the energy and turning the wrist inwards. Hold the breath for few seconds and come back in normal position

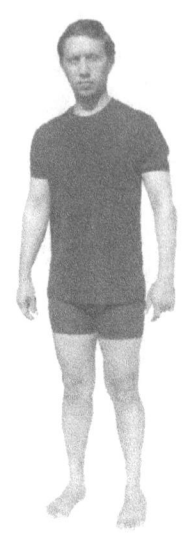

This is just an approach towards feeling of energy. It is not a conditioned way. One can make his own way because every individual is different. I will give a little idea of how to move.

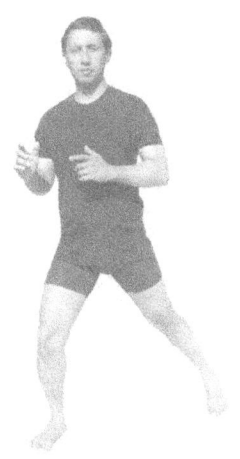

This is when you want to turn on say left side. Put more weight on your right leg take your left leg sideways toe touching to ground. Slowly turn to left side.

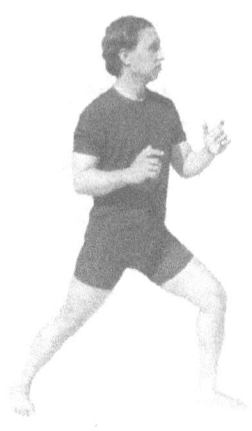

Same way turn on right side

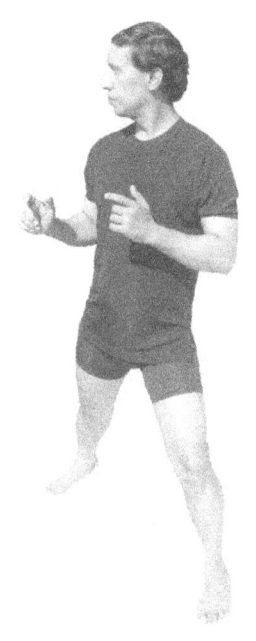

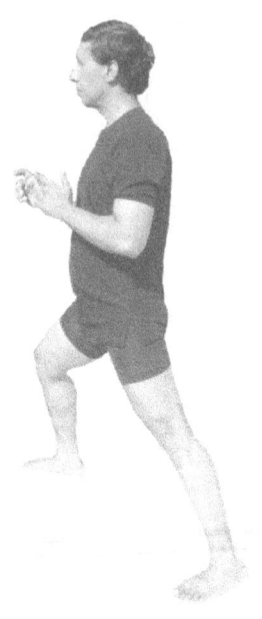

While practicing these you can initially do inhalation and exhalation alternately. When you feel comfortable you can do two times inhalation and three times exhalation. Then four times exhalation. Idea is to make exhalation double of inhalation or increase the time of exhalation. This can be done by any one old or young. Holding the breath after inhale is dangerous if you do beyond your capacity. Holding the breath after exhale is not that dangerous. Prolonged inhalation and exhalation as in ujjayi pranayama in kriya yoga gives the same effect as given by holding the breath.Further poses I am explaining about breathing process.

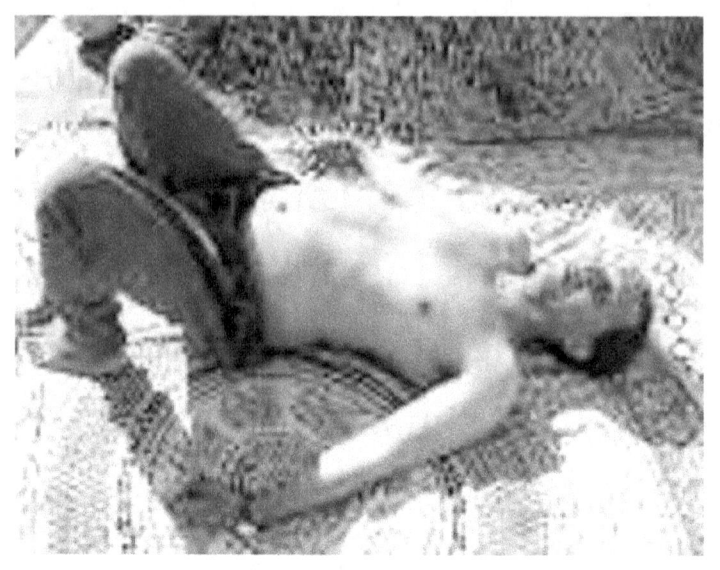

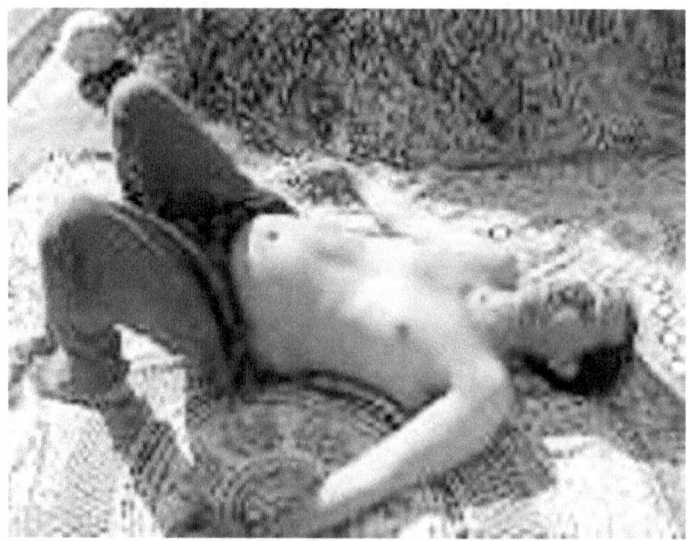

These four poses are known as tadagi mudra. Meaning lake like in the first pose inhale fully expanding the stomach .Generally if you are aware when we inhale first our stomach is protruded and then the rib cage and thoracic region finally the shoulders exhaling is in the reverse order. In this pose after inhaling and expanding the stomach exhale and push the stomach outside further and hold your nose, now let the stomach drop and go inside on its own. Keep for few seconds holding the breath and then release. This is the preparatory pose for any pose which requires abdominal lift such as Nauli or uddiyan bandh

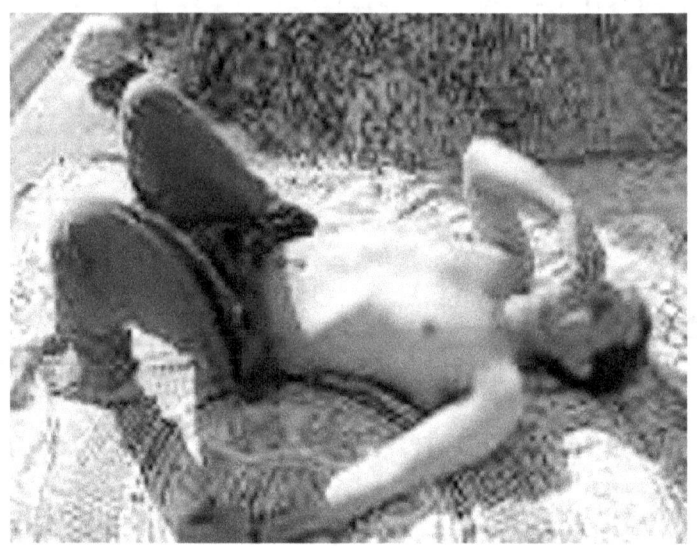

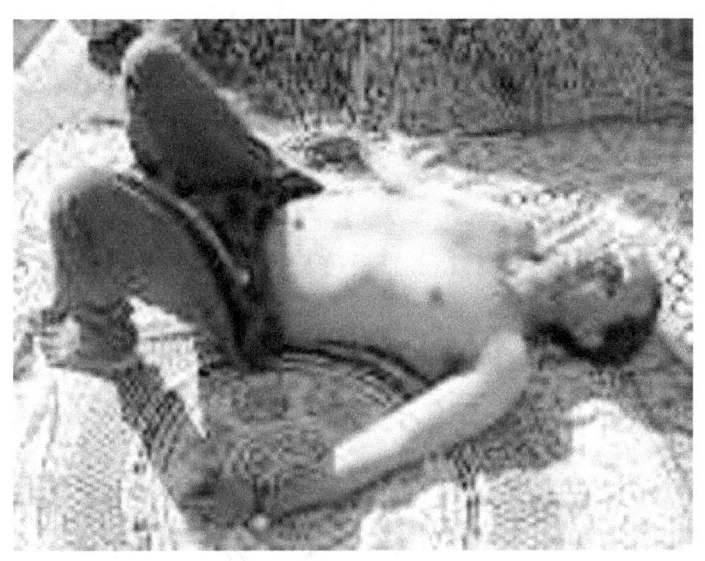

GENERAL AWARENESS OF BREATHING PROCESS

We should be aware of generally how we breath, normally people know that we breathe by expanding chest, as we don't fill in our lungs to its fullest capacity neither we expel the breath to its fullest capacity, the residual remains our body and brain both are starved and if the residual

271

remains it may be dangerous leaving body for other diseases of lungs.

So when we breathe, first the abdominal muscles are expanded then the rib cage, chest and shoulders are lifted slightly and while releasing the reverse is done, by doing this we are using abdomen and thoracic or chest breathing, by doing this lungs get the optimum amount of air removing the residual to its fullest, which prevents the lungs from any diseases.

PRANAYAMA

Prana is a vital force which is in the whole of creation, the air we breathe is not exactly the prana. Prana is subtler it is an essence or the vital force by which even the air is lively, yama means to control, so to control prana is pranayama.

Just holding breath may be dangerous, for pranayama one should go through some expert, or do it as easily as possible, we see when a person is engrossed in some work, he generally breathes very slowly, quick and uneven breathing happens at the time of anger, fear or lust. The monkey breathes at the rate of 32times a minute, a man's average breathe is 18 times a minute, the tortoise who lives for 300 years just breathes 4 times a minutes.

Prolong inhalation and exhalation as in bhramari pranayama also gives the same effect, not necessary that you hold the breath for longer time, as in kriya yoga there is no holding of breath but the effect is great, the blood is decarbonized and recharged with oxygen and the atoms of this extra oxygen are transmuted in to life current to rejuvenate the brain and spinal centre's, by stopping the accumulation of venous blood, the yogi is able to lessen or prevent the decay of the tissues.

People with high blood pressure or any other problems should consult the doctor before starting the practices.

Prana is divided into 5 pranas

PRANA: Controls respiratory systems and speech organs, activates inhalation and exhalation.

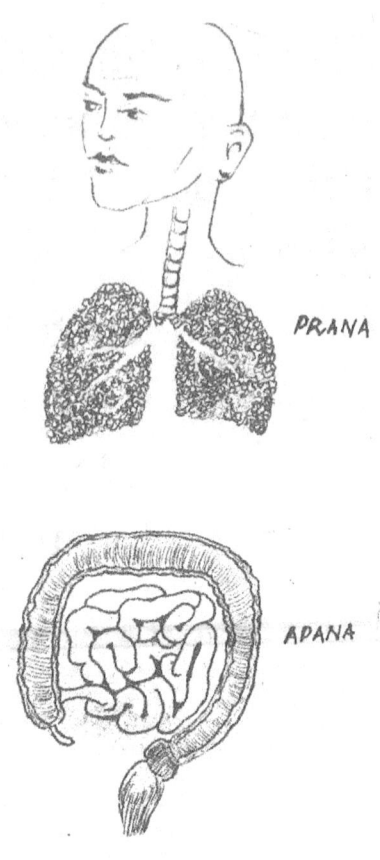

PRANA

APANA

APANA: Located below the naval region and activates expulsions and helps eliminations

SAMANA: Activates and controls

the digestive system, it is concerned with the region between the heart and the naval and helps assimilation of the nutrients

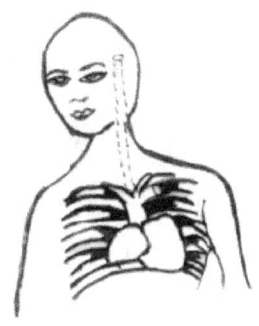

UDANA: Dwells in the thoracic cavity and controls the intake of air and food, helps metabolism.

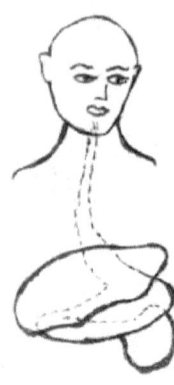

VYANA: It is a vital force, pervading the whole body harmonizes and activates the feet, hands and other body instruments and their associated muscles, ligaments, nerves and joints

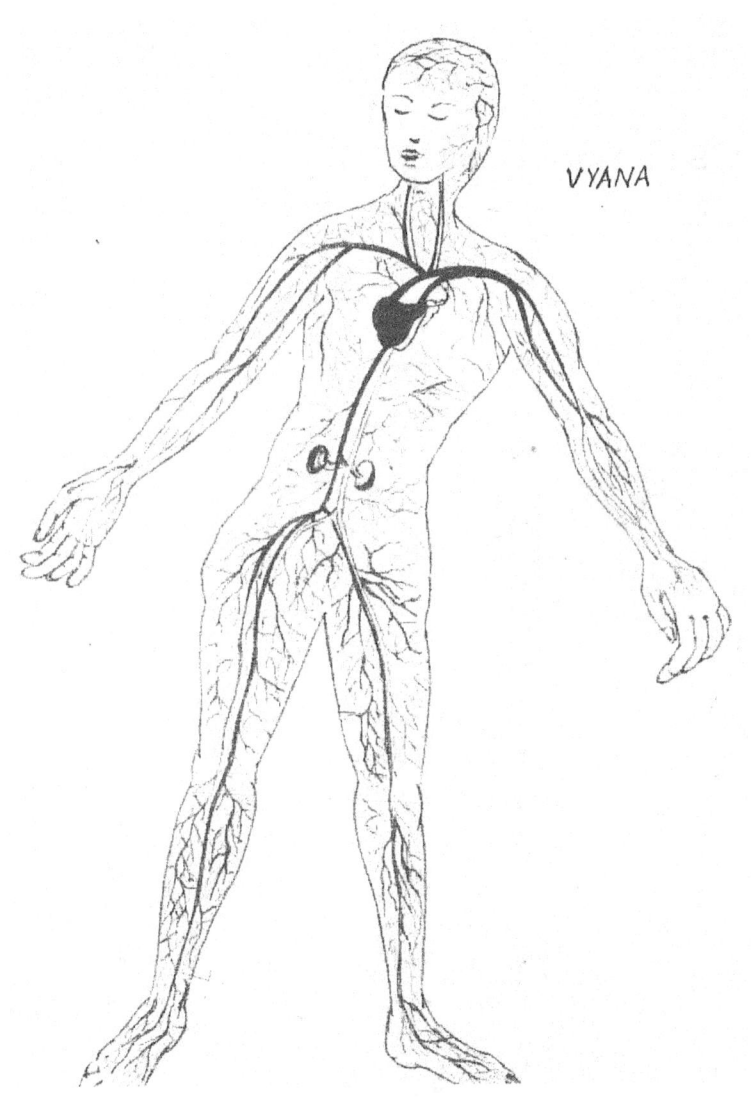

VYANA

UDDIYAN BANDHA

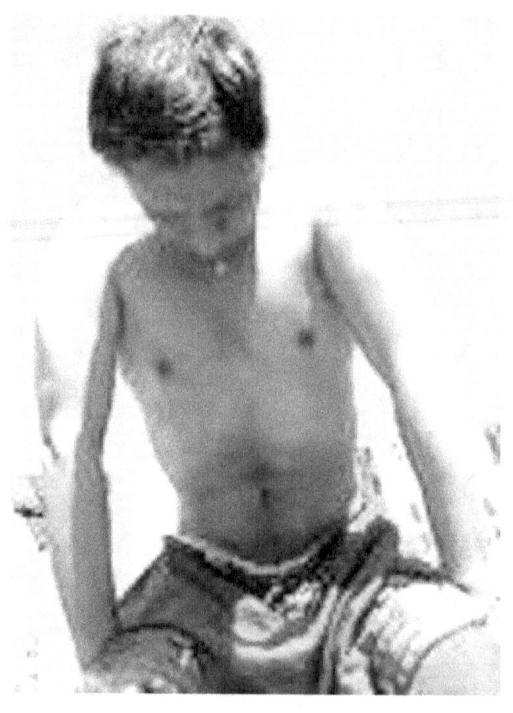

As explained earlierTadagi mudra

or lake like pose helps in performing Uddiyan bandha meaning abdominal lift.Here it is done by bending the knees.Placing the palms at mid of the thighs inhale fully by protruding stomach then exhale by pushing the stomach further as in tadagi mudra, hold the breath and let the stomach go inside.In this position while holding the breath if you start taking stomach inside and outside or moving the stomach rhythmically it is known as AGNISAR KRIYA which is preparotary pose for Nauli the churning of abdominal muscles.This control wind bile and and mucus which results in rejuvenating the system.

NAULI

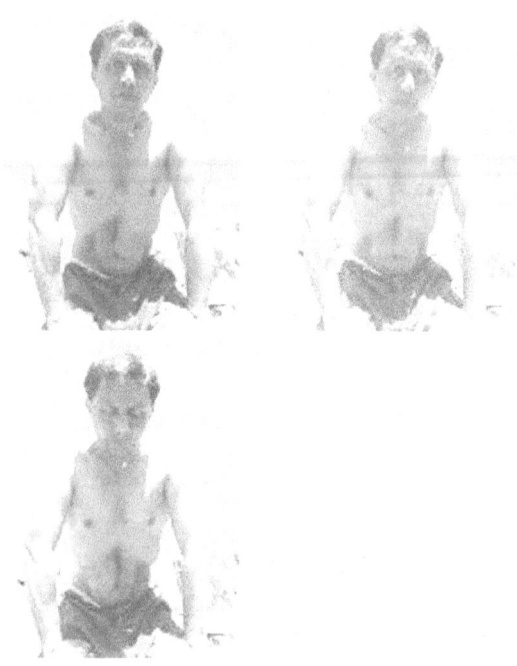

When you will put pressure on one of the palms kept on the mid of the thigh. One side of the intestinal muscles will be affected and protruded. Practice same with the other side so other side of muscles will be protruded. If you put pressure on both the palms only the mid portion will come out. With the help of both the palms moving alternately you can make the muscles move circularly which is known as NAULI.

JANUSHIRASANA

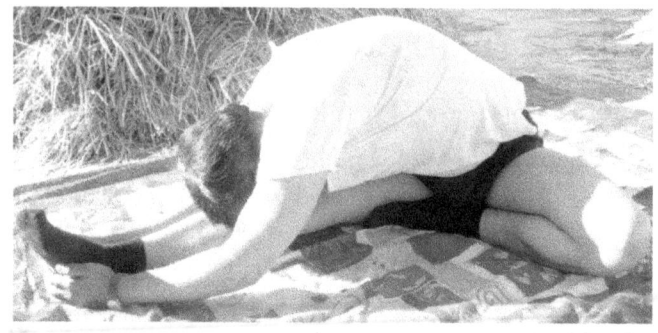

This pose is known as
janushirasana in hathayoga. In
kriyoga it is performed as
Mahamudra.It prolongs the time of
cell disintegration thus keeps the
person rejuvenating and full of
vigor. Bend any one of your knee

and place your feet at inner thigh the other foot straight. Exhale take stomach inside this is known as uddiyan bandh and hold the breath .Contract the area between anus and scrotum this is known as mula bandha.Touch your chin towards chest this is known as jalandhar bandha, try to hold your extended foot as easy as possible and touch your head to the knee. Slowly release the breath and relax. These bandhas or locks have profound pschophysiological effect in your endocrinal system. They are infinitely better than modern exercises. These were used by

Aryans who were believed to come from outer space. They were highly evolved beings. It depends on the reader if he wants he can take or leave it. Because even prolonging life span has no meaning if you don't know thyself. These bandhas or locks can be done in conjunction with mudras for better effects. Science of mudras is an ancient subject put in front of mankind by the rishis for the better and healthy living, according to them the secret of health and rejuvenation lies in hands.

Mudras are performed with the help of fingers, these are

condensed in the traditional philosophical dances, also were performed in martial arts and Indian rituals.

Our body is made up of five basic element earth, water, fire, air and space, in order to keep the body healthy any disturbances caused in the body can be cured by performing these mudras and bandhas.

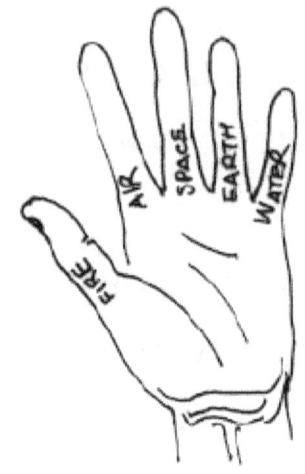

Five fingers of the palm controls five basic elements thumb—fire, index finger—air, middle finger—space, ring finger—earth, small finger—water.

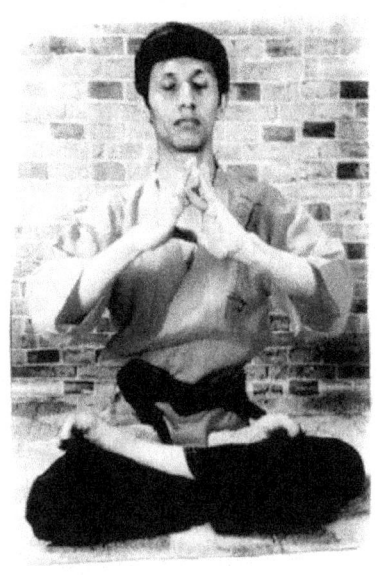

Cow posture, fingers of both the palms should be placed in a way that both the ring finger touches the tip of the last smaller fingers, crossing each other, then middle fingers touching the tips of the index fingers, as shown.

Benefits in memory stimulating and improves the memory power.

Dhyan mudra

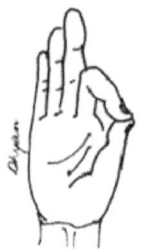

Touch the thumb with the index finger, these mudras can be performed in any easy postures.

Benefits: It is the most important mudra used for meditation, helps in increasing brain power, prevents mental disorders, mental tensions.

Prana mudra

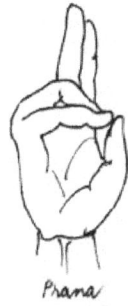

Prana

Bend the little and ring fingers so that, their tips touch the tip of thumb as shown.

Benefits for improving eye power increases life force ki or prana

Linga mudra

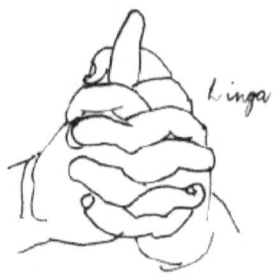

Entangle the fingers of both the palms keeping either of the thumbs erect.

It benefits in case of cold and bronchial infections.

Vayu mudra

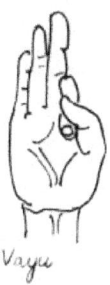

Vayu

Touch the index finger at the base of the thumb that is mounting of Venus as shown.

Benefits, it prevents rheumatism and purifies blood.

Sunya mudra

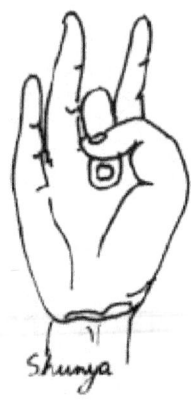

Shunya

Keep the middle finger at the top of the Venus as shown in fig and press lightly with the thumb.

Benefits, it affects the person who is weak in hearing, also beneficial in vertigo.

Varun mudra

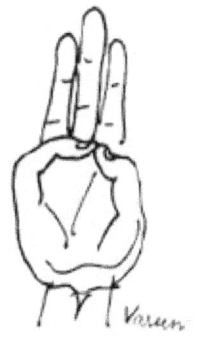

Touch the tips of thumb and little finger together as shown.

Benefits in gastro intestinal problems, helps skin to become smoother.

Prithvi mudra

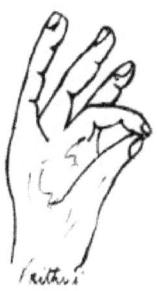

Touch the ring finger to the thumb as shown.

Benefits in maintaining the balance of earth element in our body, strives for eradicating physical weakness.

Sun mudra

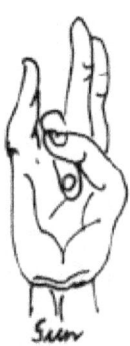

Bend ring finger so as on its outer side on second fold, you can press with the thumb as shown.

It benefits in weight reduction and removal of fats in the body.

Yoga mudra

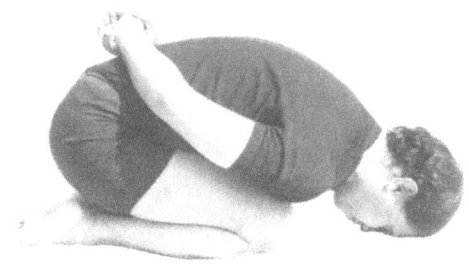

Sit in padmasana or vajrasana grasp one wrist behind the back with the other hand, slowly bending the upper body, bring the head to the floor, touch the forehead to the floor, remain in the position, slowly assume the starting pose and relax.

This is preventive for abdominal ailments and vertebrae related problems.

Kaki Mudra

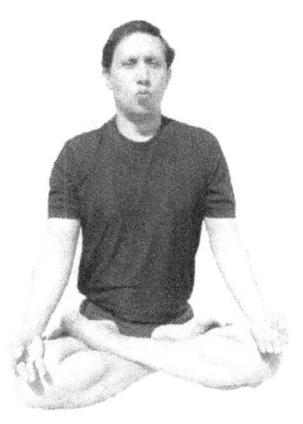

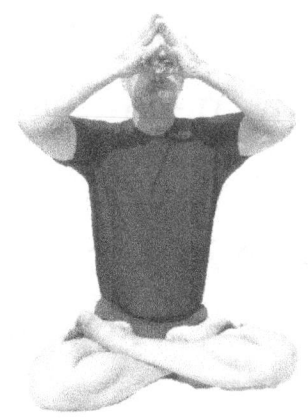

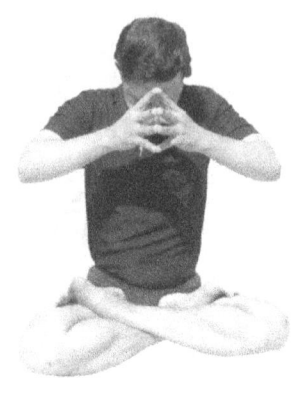

I

n this mudra the lips are pursed resembling a crows beak, can be done in any meditative pose, this mudra is very good for overall development of the face, by regular practicing cheeks become red. It is a age defying balm.

Close your both the nostrils with both the thumbs, fingers touching their tips, start inhaling through the lips, open your eyes while inhaling, after inhaling, expand both your cheeks, touch your chin to the chest and hold your breath as per your capacity.

After performing those bring your head to the normal position, slowly open your eyes & release your breath through nose.

Simha mudra

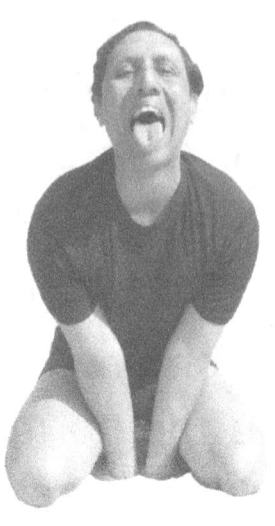

This is a symbol of lion, practicing this mudra reduces the wrinkles from the face, effects are much better if done in conjunction with jiva bandha, tongue lock taking the tongue to the upper palate of the mouth and also stretching it outside as shown.

Controls enlargement of tonsils, stabilizes blood pressure.

Sit on vajrasana on the heels, open up the knees resting the body on arms, tilt the head backward, extend the tongue by opening the mouth open, eyes wide gazing at eyebrows exhale producing a sound as it comes exhaling through open mouth.

Vajroli mudra

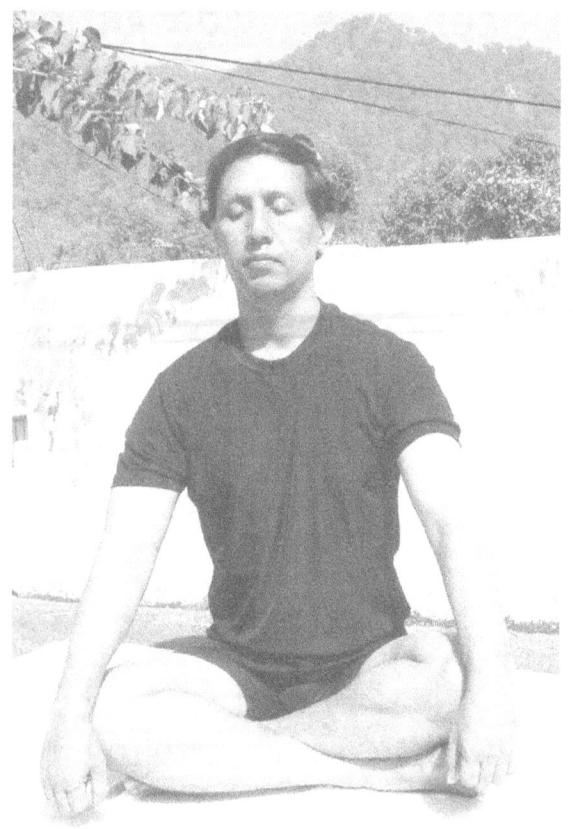

Practice of vajroli mudra controls the vajra nadi by which sexual energy is controlled and semen retention power is increased. This posture is sukhasana easy cross leg pose.

Sit in any meditative pose or sukhasana, put your awareness in sex organs for males, contract the penis and pull upward for females contract the clitoris, lower vaginal muscles and urethra and pull upwards. Hold for few seconds and release. Initially one tends to contract all the muscles of anus, penis and the place anus ant testes. But you should try to segregate all three of them place between testes and anus. But with practice you can segregate them

Ashwini mudra

This is preventive in the case of piles, sit in any meditative pose or sukhasana put your awareness at the muscles of anus contract the anus and release, do it as easily as possible without straining. This can be done in conjunction with pawanmuktasana for prevention of piles.

Moola bandha

Is usefull in both the purposes to attain celibacy and to prevent the sexual problems, it takes the sexual energy upward for spiritual development or downward to enhance marital relations.

It controls the life force consequently psychosomatic degeneration is controlled increases vitality, also increases the sexual retention power, and should not be practice in case of absence of periods for females.

Moolabandha may be practiced at the time of pregnancy for increasing the elasticity of the muscles also after child birth, along with vajroli mudra and aswini mudra for restoring the muscles and controlling the neuro muscular system, it generates excessive sexual energy, prevents hernia, and controls testosterone secretions.

Sit in any meditative pose or sukhasana, put your awareness at the place between the scrotum and anus, contract that place and draw the muscles upward, initially it is difficult to draw only muscles of that area, all three gets contracted but in due course of time it happens.

KAPALBHATI PRANAYAMA

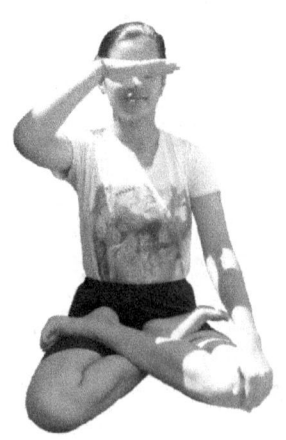

Before explaining Kapalbhati let me explain half kapalbhati or also known as suddhi kriya.Close one nostril with your thumb and expell or exhale through other nostril taking the lower abdomen inside.Do not force after doing one stroke wait for the air to come inside naturally then go for other stroke.Can be done ten times through each nostril do three sets or as per your capacity.If same is done with both the nostrils it is known as kapalbhatti.

CHECK This I am writing specifically because it applies to all asanas and pranayamas.Akso I have seen many people performing incorrect.

If you fall short of breath after performing then it is done wrongly.

Sit in any meditative postures or sukhasana, expel your breath forcefully through your nose taking your stomach inwards, do it initially for 50-60 breaths then relax after some time, perform moolabandha and do the same practice. Gradually increase it to thousand exhales.

Benefits: it prepares you for meditation, purifies frontal region of brain as the name suggests kapal bhati, it shines the forehead, beneficial in the case of cerebral thrombosis.

BHASTRIKA PRANAYAMA

Sit in any meditative posture or sukhasana perform moola bandha.As you perform moolabandha your lower abdomen is locked. Now you can move upper abdomen keeping the body steady, hands rooted or kept on knees as in kapalbhatti breathe rapidly. Inhaling and exhaling rapidly using upper abdomen. Initially do it slowly so that counts can be increased after around fifty or hundred counts. One count is one inhalation and exhalation, exhale fully then inhale through right nostril hold the breath touch the chin to the chest and retain as easily as possible.If you have done moolabandha also while retaining the breath then before exhalation release moolabandha. Exhale through left nostril. If you feel thisis difficult practice. The easier way is by inhaling and exhaling by concentrating on chest, do not move the shoulders. Hands rooted at knees by this also you will feel you are moving upper abdominal muscles gradually when you understand this you can perform as explained earlier.

Benefits: it removes the impurities from the lungs, benefits in asthma, tuberculosis

BHRAMARI PRANAYAMA

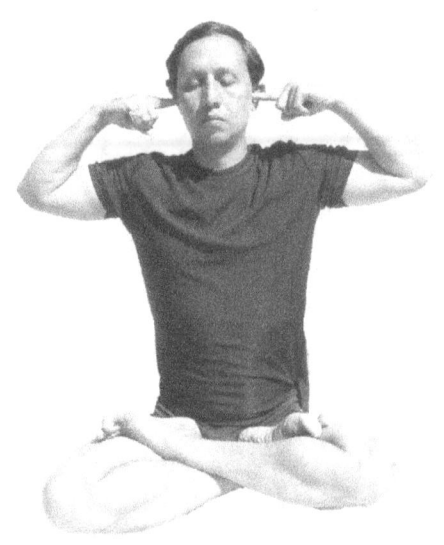

Sit in any meditative pose or sukhasana, spine erect plug both the ears with index fingers. Mouth closed, take breath through the nostrils, hold it for a second and start releasing the breath from nose producing m m m sound while mouth closed slowly release the hands and relax.

Benefits in blood pressure problems, develops the sound quality or the voice, relieves mental tension.

ANULOM VILOM PRANAYAMA

Sit in any meditative pose or sukhasana, spine erect.Closing the left nostril exhale through right nostril and then inhale through the same right nostril.Hold the breath for few seconds then exhale through left nostril hold for few seconds.Further inhale through the same left nostril and exhale through right nostril.This completes one round of anulom vilom.One can increase as per his capacity.It is very good for balancing the system and improvement of eyesight

It is more of thinking which puts

the technique in proper.

You have to think before doing the technique and you have be aware of that thought while performing to be vigil and you have to be aware or recollect after you have done.

Let me tell you about a debate which affects the thinking as a whole giving after effects as a results, in which I to happen to Participate, the topic was India should or should not make an Atom bomb, talk either for or against. I talked for; India should make an atom bomb. When EmperorAsokalaid down his weapons and took a woe that he will never use weapons', the empire was finished. He became a Buddha follower. The important thing here was not winning or losing or leaving or accepting, what was important was the psychological effect

A combine of martial art and yoga does not advocate self renunciation. On the contrary it teaches 'pragmatism',

Its meaning is self improvement which can come in handy in material life. This concept will become clear if one were to draw an analogy from what the Great

Emperor Asoka did,

Asoka renounced all weapons and embraced Buddhist Philosophy. There is no denying the noble intentions, but the fact remains that the spiritual ethos that is sought is not applicable to the common man or the material world where there is a need to constantly be on the alert and keep a vigil on the surrounding. Touching on the present day relevance of this analogy one can entertain debates on whether India should be a Nuclear power or not? The simple answer to this comes – Yes. We need to defend our frontiers for the well being of the present or future generations. There are no escaping facts. Similarly, the martial art yoga combine will teach you to face reality in life rather than runaway from it, but remembering non violence at our innermost core. We recollect from GuruGobindsingh's time, he being the perfect master fought for the right cause, because of the cruelty of Muslimking. Once at the time of war one of his men was feeding water to a Muslim fighter also. To which Hindus objected and complained. Master asked to the person why he was doing so, the person replied sir, didn't you say at Satsanga all human beings come from the same light. Master said all right you can feed water to both. This is the learning of pure thinking. That is how In Greece, Plato abolished dance from the ideal republic, whose citizens were capable of pure thought and had no need of sensory images. In Book 7 of the laws, though, Plato was concerned with a more practical social structure, here he admitted two forms of art, gymnastic and theatrical dance they were aid to health beauty and reflecting the harmony of a noble and ordered mind: their virtues were simplicity, measure and symmetry. Aristotle preferred to stress the closeness to drama "even the dancer like the actor, imitate men's characters as well as what they do and suffer. The analogy to music and drama would be used for centuries thereafter.

The word Yoga and Aurveda are derived from Athaarvaveda

The word Yunj means to join the soul with the supreme soul. The adepts were using the combination of both, to keep their mind and body fit for the meeting of finite to infinite.

Yoga is derived from Maharishi Patanjali's sutra a 'Yogas chitta vritti nirodha'. Many personalities have defined this sloka from sutra no 2 Chapter 1 as 'supression of modification of mind as Yoga '. According to me, Mind is not chitta to which Patanjali is reffering, chitta is still subtler and is consciousness. Tendency of the consciousness is related with the mind. When I see an object, the information goes to the mind and in turn creates impressions on the consciousness which affects and creates vritties on consciousness. Vritties can be called as cessations and can be compared to ripples forming in a pond, when a stone is thrown. These cessations forming on the consciousness are to be calm down so the meaning of the sloka is calming down of cessation of consciousness is Yoga.

By constantly practicing with the individuals of different types, I started understanding the words used by the masters "to teach one to be skillfull is easy, to teach him his own attitude is rather difficult" and that is where the mastery of the teaching lies. Education word is derived from a Latin Educare means 'to educe' or to unfold the talents of the individual. Attitudes, skill, philosophy, ideocyncracies all should be understood to bring out the individuals or students hidden talents. It is required because we are all working for increasing the awareness and the upliftment of human beings. So any method yogic or scientific should be used.At times when I used to go to meet some yogis, I used to think because they are great I can see Aura. But at times I used to see Aura behind anybody. This, I was surprised when I read about the same thing in kirlian' s photography, kirlian' s a husband and a wife team, a great scientists and philosopher from soviet Union, invented a specially sensitive film camera which can see things which eyes can not see. His photographs showed Auras around   all the human beings, animals and Trees and when he took a photpgraph of a dead person he found that the Aura was missing. Just six months before the death, the Aura was missing and I came to know that I have increased my sensitivity by meditation. If one is angry or sad the Aura will be small, if he is peaceful or silent

The Aura will be bigger. This Aura is like an electromagnetic field which can be measured and photographed. Even the

Vedas state that every object is consisting of a pranic field which appears as an encompassing mass of Light. This kirlian's photography is a great invention. Modern science has devised instruments like Electro Encephalograph which can be of aid to any art. This is an amplifer system which can detect electrical activities occurring within the brain. These are picked up by the means of electrods, fixed to the sides of the head. These electrical patterns can be recorded on a graph by a pen recorder, which will indicate the type of wave being emitted. The shape of the wave, serve as an indicator for reading the state of mind. By knowing one's brain wave activity, conscious steps can be taken to reach to the desired state. Researchers show that all the body processes can be controlled; this is what has been said by the yogis thousands of years ago. Yet, it is recently been taken seriously by modern scientist. These scientific instruments popularly known as bio feed back system. Specifically for the people who are less interested in meditation and much more in scientific explanation and sciences. Yogic philosophy extends far beyond the range of vision of medical science. Scientific work in a great way compliments yoga because some people are so insensitive that they lack the ability to feel whether they are relaxed or tensed. Martial artist Bruce Lee can be the supreme example of this sentence.

He started from the wing Chun system, where the ability to sense

and feel dominates, and from
there he developed himself to the
state of understanding his frame of
mind and he tried to break every
sort of conditioning. He also
referred to Indian philosopher J
Krishnamurti. If today people are
not much aware, the reason is
misunderstanding of what
education is, it is not the amount
of information that gets
accumulated in your brain,
undigested, for education is to
learn and be aware and takes the
awareness to such an extent so as
to understand the universality of
the spirit. I would like to quote Sir

Albert Einstein. He says "A University is a place in which the universality of human spirit finds self expression. Unfortunately the universities of Europe today are the nurseries of chauvinism of blind intolerance". What Einstein said of European Universities is applicable to almost all Universities found in the world so far. If education is not understood in that light of universality of the spirit, the peace extinguishes and such education becomes clinical.

Consequently competition comes into play and the real knowing lags behind. Needless to say in the heat of competition, the process of learning and knowing is hampered. That's why according to me art is where, competition is not involved and inner being of individual flows.Vajramukti is such a form. If we divide our whole existence into seven parts it will be astonishing to know that we are aware of only one part out of seven about our relationship with the environment, $1/7^{th}$ in control of ourselves and $1/7^{th}$ of what we are physically, mentally and metaphysically capable of living. But if we develop this by constantly being aware of our self with our tools that is body and its parts, this awareness which neither rejects nor selects , a choice less awareness. This is a state of moving meditation and in this awareness we shall be using the naval region as the center of action, which is also said to be 7 cm or some movement arts or dancers believe 3 inches below the navel beneath, which at the coccyx rests the kundalini power or serpent power. By using this region as the point of center of action, performance capacity increases to maximum with minimum fatigue. The ideal goal is one has to become an observer of the interplay which can also put one in contact with the eternal reality. This state of becoming an observer and witnessing one's own act & being choicelessly aware is known as 'shakshibhavana'. After moving meditation, comes sitting meditation, which is called za-zen in martial arts circle. It is surprising to know that 'Zen' word extensively used in martial arts circles, has got its roots in India. Specifically in Sanskrit language the root word is 'Dhyan'. Gautam Buddha after his enlightment started using word from his native language Pali that is 'Zhan'.

When Bodhidharma went to china to spread Buddhism, the word changed in 'Chan' and finally in Japan it became 'Zen'.

The interesting part is, from movement one precedes to non movement. That is what Za-zen is 'Sitting meditation'. It happened with me once after doing movements with breathing. I sat down in a lotus posture and started thinking, whatever the thought was, good or bad, and then I started witnessing the thoughts, they disappeared within an instant, surprisingly. I was then taken over by a light which I could see in my inner sky. When I started concentrating on the light, my body consciousness was losing. This was the first time I clearly felt that I am not the body. I sat there for five hours but it was as if just five minutes had passed.Equivalent word for Zen in English is meditation. It condenses of concentration and contemplation. These two words are applicable at initial stages. But all concentration contemplation and meditation is not Dhayana because dhayan happens you cannot do deliberately.Concentration is withdrawing of attention from the objects of distraction and then focusing of that recalled attention upon one thing at a time or it is an art of focusing all the powers of attention upon a single point or focusing mind on one thing or one thought. Contemplation is focusing mind not only on thought but by the stream of thought confined to one subject.In concentration mind focuses on one thought. In contemplation mind focuses from one thought to s stream of thought on one particular subject. And in meditation mind meditates. Dhyan happens when one goes beyond the mind. That is why Upanishads say "their neither speech goes nor the mind, from there the knowing of that one truth starts, we call it by some name you can call it by any name, it is beyond name and form, it is the experience"..But still one can say meditation is the concentration and contemplation combined and used to know the indwelling truth, within ourselves and in turn the supreme reality. Whatever your vocation may be a martial artist, medicine man, business man, house holder etc., you can increase your efficiency by hundred percent by the regular deep practice of meditation

PREVENTION & REHABILITATION

Body and mind are inseparably related with each other. When there is too much anxiety. It affects the physical as well as the mental state. Medical tests have shown that patients suffering from Neuroses, High blood pressure, mental tension, anxiety has got a high level of lactate compared to when they are calm & tranquil. Meditation is the easy and natural method of reducing the lactate level, by practicing, positive influence on the blood pressure can be noticed, pressure drops during and after meditation. During meditation, sympathetic system activities are reduced resulting in the decrease of the constriction of the blood vessels & hence greater flow of blood, which benefits the one who meditates. To prove the value of meditation one might easily say that your grasping power increases amazingly, you start learning easily and quickly, but this statement is coming out of resistance .Meditation is to calm down. Once you imply the word easily and quickly, the resistance is the very word, the time is doubled and the stress develops. There is nothing as mind controlling because in the subtler state, there is no mind. You can use the word consciousness, but is there any degree in consciousness? It is up to the one who experiences.

CASE OF ASTHAMA

One's one businessman told me that he is getting an asthmatic attack. I made him sit in vajrasana and pull his hand upward relax the head at floor which started his abdominal breathing and he was relieved. Asthma is a chronic psychosomatic disease, meaning those diseases' where in emotional psychic factors are closely related.

In asthma the breathing passage becomes constricted, as a result the individual experiences severe difficulty while breathing. The air we inhale, moves through trachea, the bronchi and then enters cells of the lungs, these narrow bronchi are constricted due to reason such as mucus. It results in difficulty in breathing.

The postures which are beneficial I am giving here. Breathing should be normal do not hold the breath.

ASTHMA

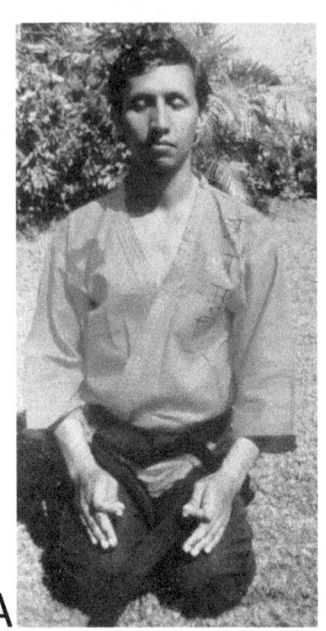

1   VAJRASANA

2   SHUDDHI KRIYA

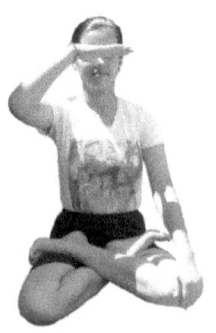

3   SUPTA VAJRASANA

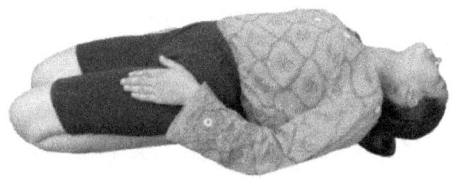

4   BHUJANGASANA

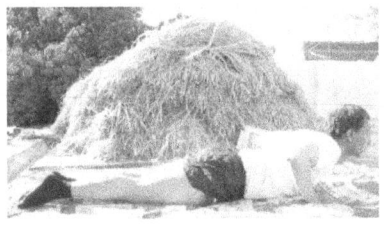

5 SHALABHASANA

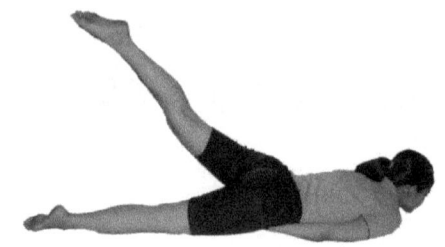

6 DHANURASANA

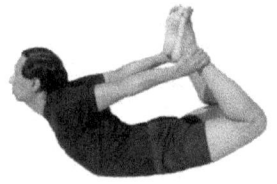

7 MAKARASANA

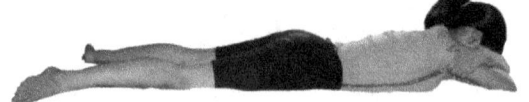

8   MATSYASANA

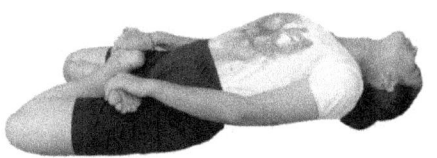

9   TADAGI MUDRA

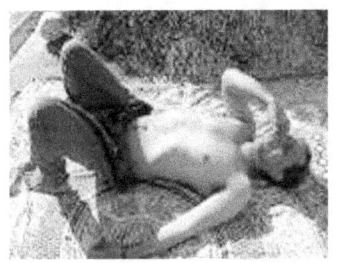

10 SIMHA MUDRA

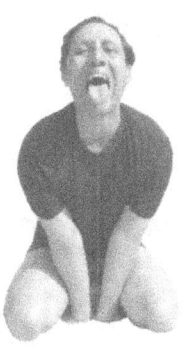

11 SHAVASANA

DIABETES

Prevention and control of Diabetes

Also used for prevention and rehabilitation. In diabetes the sugar level is elevated in the blood, it happens by dis easing The body's system of assimilating and utilizing glucose, which affects other vital organs of the body, pancreas,liver,kidney & complicates the body functioning. It is mainly a stress related disorder.

Postures for prevention and rehabilitation are as given below.

1VAJRASANA

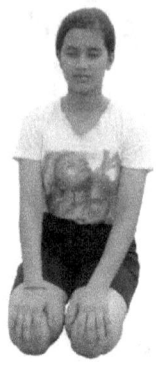

2 SHUDDHIKRIYA

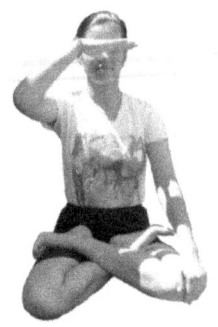

3 JANU SHIRASANA

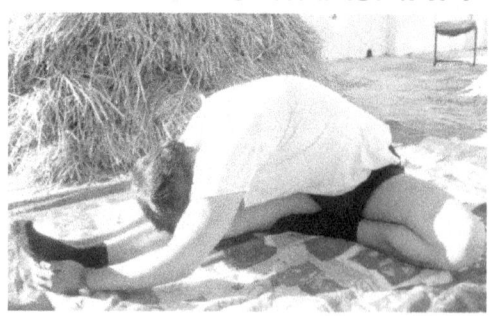

4 PASCHIMOTTANASANA

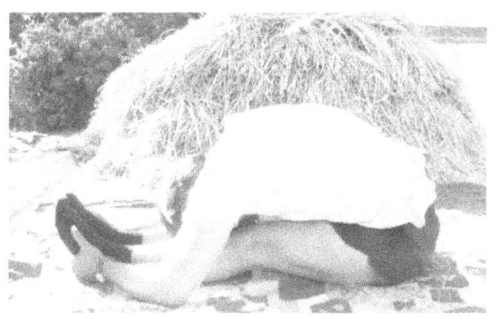

5BHUJANGASANA

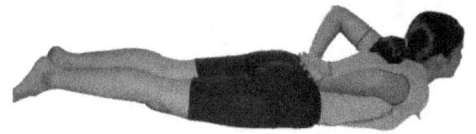

6 MATSYASANA

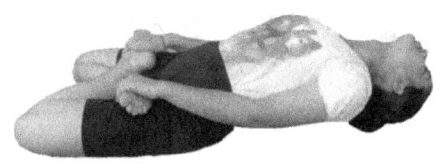

7 SARVANGASANA

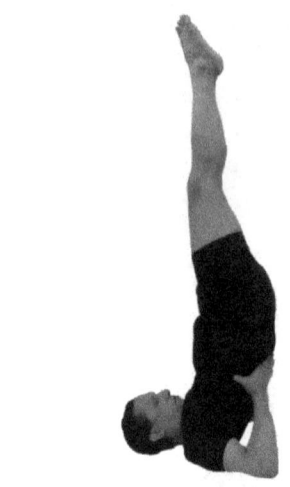

8   HALASANA

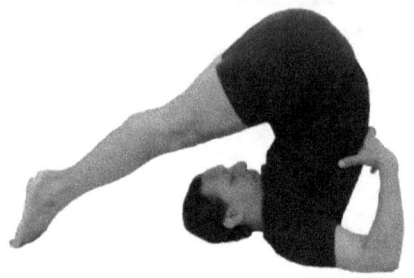

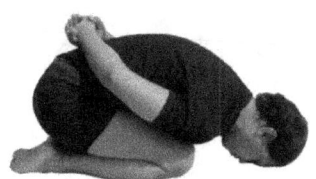

10 UJJAYI PRANAYAMA

11 SHAVASANA

HIGH AND LOW BLOOD PRESSURE

The main factor affecting the rhythmic fluctuation or pulsations of the heart is stressful lifestyle. If it is an emergency medicinal help must be taken also whenever require but as prevention and rehabilitation these poses will be of great help for high blood pressure practice Pawanmuktasana and Ujjayi pranayama for low blood pressure surya namaskar, bhastrika pranayama and kapalbhatti.

PAVANMUKTASANA

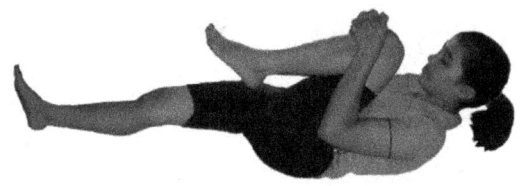

SAVASANA

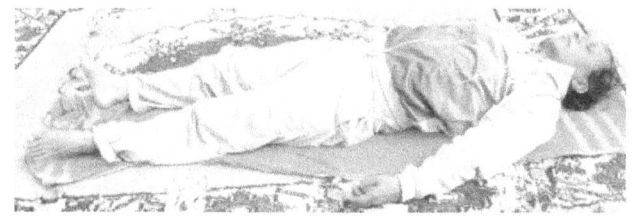

UJJAYIPRANAYAMA

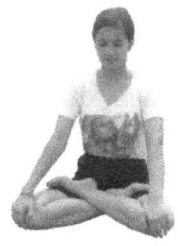

LOW-BLOOD PRESSURE

SURYANAMASKARA

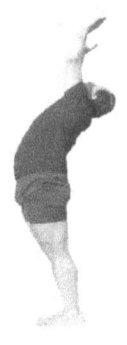

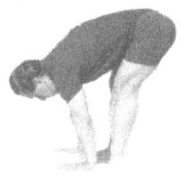

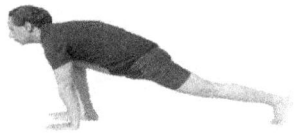

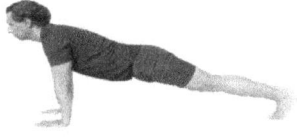

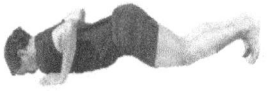

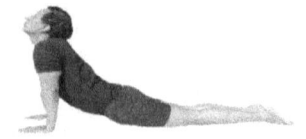

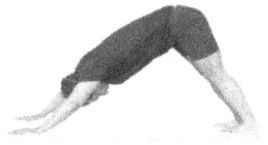

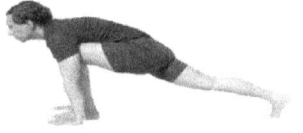

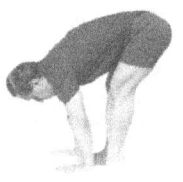

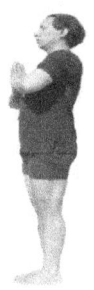

Kapalbhati pranayama

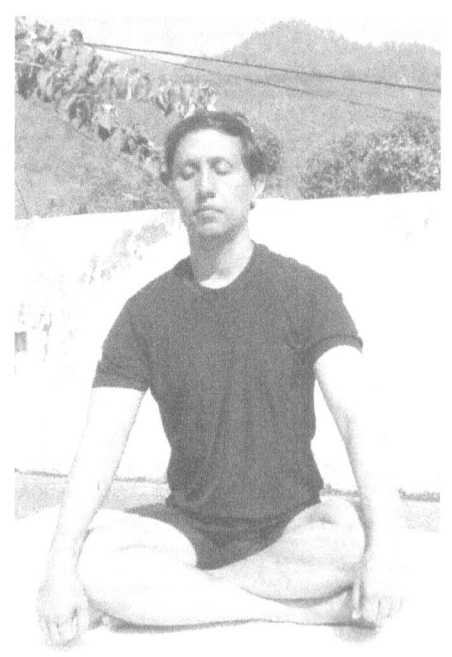

Sit in any meditative postures or sukhasana, expel your breath forcefully through your nose taking your stomach inwards, do it initially for 50-60 breaths then relax after some time, perform Moolabandha and do the same practice. Gradually increase it to thousand exhales.

Benefits: it prepares you for meditation, purifies frontal region of brain as the name suggests kapal bhati, it shines the forehead, beneficial in the case of cerebral thrombosis.

BHASTRIKA PRANAYAMA

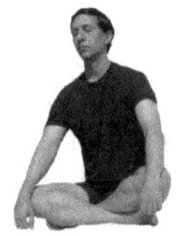

Sit in any meditative posture or sukhasana perform Moola bandha. As you perform Moolabandha your lower abdomen is locked. Now you can move upper abdomen keeping the body steady, hands rooted or kept on knees as in kapalbhatti breathe rapidly. Inhaling and exhaling rapidly using upper abdomen. Initially do it slowly so that counts can be increased after around fifty or hundred counts. One count is one inhalation and exhalation, exhale fully then inhale through right nostril hold the breath touch the chin to the chest and retain as easily as possible. If you have done Moolabandha also while retaining the breath then before exhalation release Moolabandha. Exhale through left nostril. If you find it difficult to perform the easier way is by inhaling and exhaling by concentrating on chest. Do not move the shoulder. Hands rooted at knees by this also you will feel you are moving upper abdominal muscles gradually when you understand this you can perform as explained earlier.

Benefits: it removes the impurities from the lungs, benefits in asthma, tuberculosis. Awareness and relaxation is the key factor in Vajramuktiyoga. It's an art work slowly practiced and developed so that the awareness takes care of nervous system changing the patterns of function and structure of the body.Artists from any field can understand this concept.

.

Surya namaskar in detail

This is also very important for females, it will make their breasts firm, remove extra fats from the buttocks, will make their legs shapely as in other exercises they may develop their calf muscles as mens, this will not happen while practicing surya namaskaras salutations to sun flexibility and strength both will be achieved.

It removes acne and clears the complexion because the impurities and toxins are thrown away from the body, the body of old king of aundh at the age of 110 was like a youth, by regular performing of suryanamaskars.

In todays modern, fast life, we don't have time for deep breathing exercise, generally, our mind is engaged in some thought, consequently the breathing becomes short, for females the situation is even worst, due to the better psychological conditioning done by media, they are attracted towards faster exercising clubs they join fast and leave fast and if continued mental stress develops.

Surya namaskar is such ancient yogic movement, which enables you to breathe and it powerfully influences your endocrinal system which controls the body functioning and makes it better.

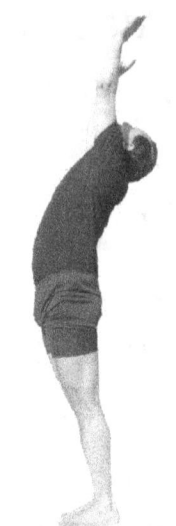

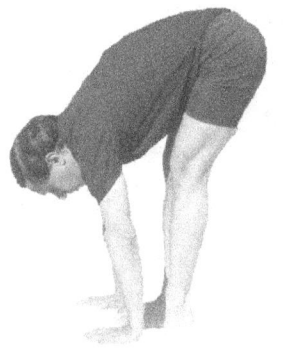

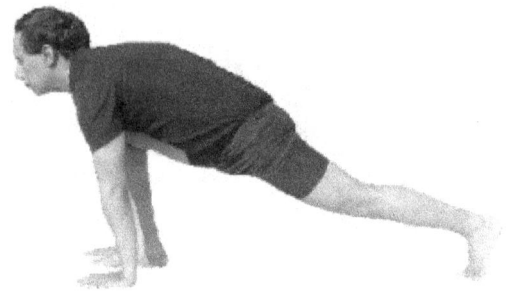

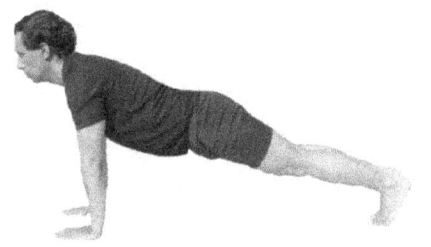

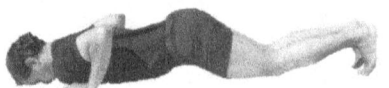

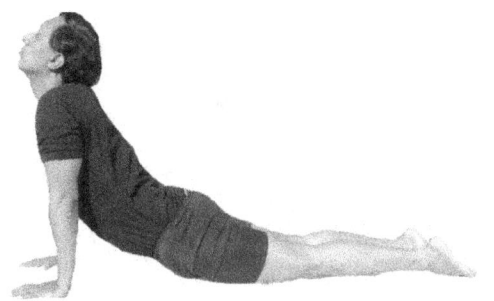

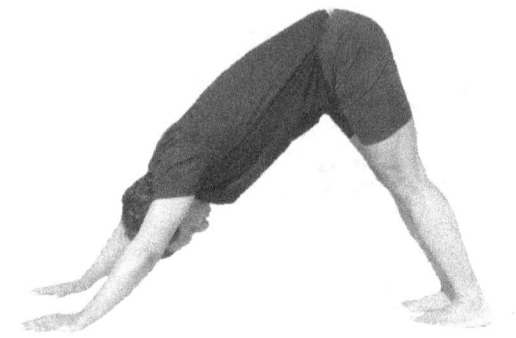

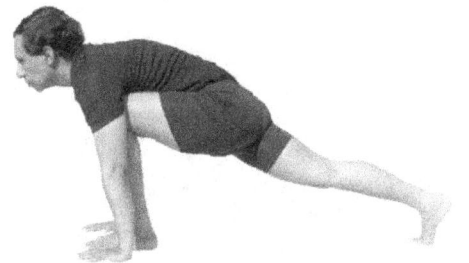

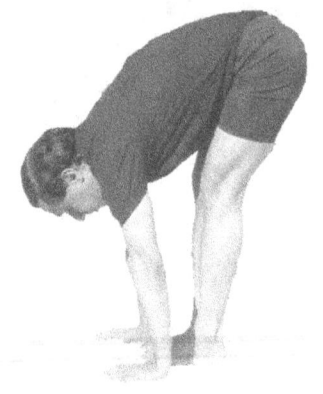

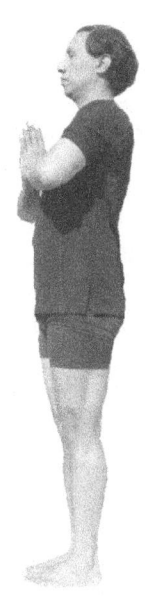

It comprises of10 steps, includes inhalation and exhalation alternately and rhythmically with the postures.

1 Stand erect feet together, raise the hands above the head

streching

and arching the back backwards, inhale.

2 Bend forward from the waist line, moving the head along with the hand; if possible try to touch the palms to the floor exhale.

3 Keep the hands rooted to the ground keeping the right foot there with knee bend, move the left foot back, look upwards arching the back inhale.

4 Take both the legs behind as in posture; hold the breath.

5 Touch the knees, palms, chest and forehead to the ground and exhale.

6 Leave the lower body on the floor, lift the upper body up and backward supported by palms, hands straight on elbows, inhale.

7 Raise your buttocks from the ground; pull your upper body back heels touching to the ground.

8 Bring the left foot in between the palms, with knee bend asin position no 3 except left foot instead of right and exhale.

9 Bring both the legs together as in position no 2 exhale.

10 Stand erect, both palms together thumb touching the sternum slowly inhale and relax.

Kapalbhati Pranayama

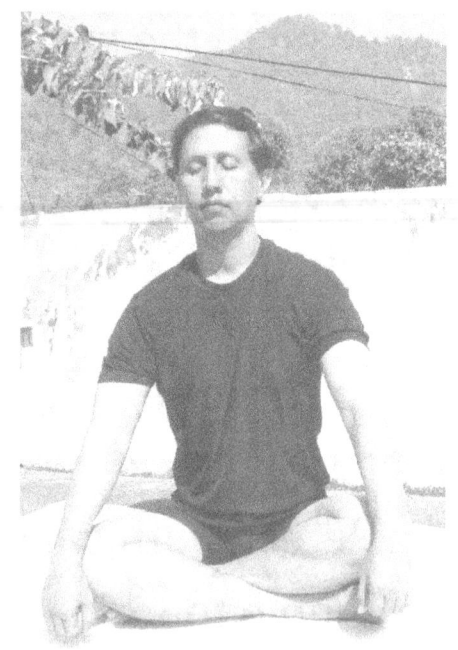

Sit in any meditative postures or
sukhasana, expel your breath

forcefully through your nose taking your stomach inwards, do for 50-60 breaths then relax after some time, perform moolabandha and do the same practice.

Benefits: it prepares you for meditation, purifies frontal region of brain as the name suggests kapal bhati, it shine the forehead, beneficial in the case of cerebral thrombosis

Bhastrika Pranayama

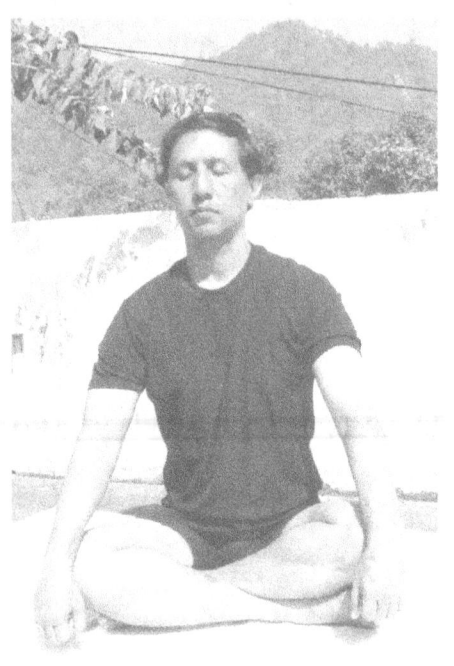

Sit in any meditative posture back straight.Be aware that your shoulders are fixed not moving, pull the middile portion between the testes and anus.This will make sure the lower abdomen is locked.

Now take deep inhalation and exhalation from chest. Do it for twenty times. As you gradually understand then you will be able to move only upper abdomen while inhaling and exhaling. You do it for twenty counts then release breath and inhale through right nostril and hold the breath as easily as possible and then release through left nostril.This makes the heart strong.

I am including my translations of Sage Patanjali's Yoga sutras

PATANJALI YOGA SUTRAS

SAMADHI PADA

1   atha yoganushasanam

Now appropriately, for the betterment of yoga practitioners, given by rishis, yoga shastra begins.

2   yogas chittivritti nirodah

The dissolution of vrittis-ripples of chitta-consciousness is yoga, chitta is made up of mana-mind, buddhi-intellect and ahamkara-ego, mana is the recording faculty, which receives impressions gathered by the senses. Buddhi is the discriminative faculty which classifies these impressions and reacts to them, ahamkara is the ego sense which claims these impressions as its own and stores them, and here vrittis are taken as ripples forming in the pond. Pond is compared to consciousness-chitta, mind is the recording faculty, a field where thought and emotion function together, it is result of sense perception, by this thought emotive activities it gives rise to tendencies which are also called as vrittis or may be called as habits of the mind; these habits become centres of reaction formed in the mind. Yoga may also be called as the state of mind completely free from all reactive tendencies.

3 *tada drastuh svarupeavasthanam*

By dissolution of the vrittis of chitta, the jivatman is established is his own nature.

4 *vritti sarupyamitaratra*

Other than those moments when he is not in the state of yoga, he remains identified with the thought waves in the mind.

5 *vrttayah panchatayah klishta aklishta*

Vrittis are of five types, divided into two klishta that includes avidhya, which is material knowledge which puts an individual into karmic etanglement, aklishta which takes you to realization or liberation, moksha.

6   *pramana viparya vikalpa nidra smrtayah*

Pramana- tool for factual knowledge, viparya-illusive knowledge, vikalpa-imagination or fancy, without any factual basis, nidra-sleep, smriti-memory these are klishta vrittis.

7   *pratyaksa anumana agamaha pramanani*

The pramana vrittis are of three type's pratyaksa anumana and agama that is sensorial cognition, inference and authority mainly the vedas and other scriptures.

8   viparyaya mithyajnanama tad rupa pratistham

When you don't understand the thing as it is or understand it as something else, this is illusory knowledge or viparyavritti.

9   sabda jnana anupati vastu sunyo vikalpah

by word knowledge if one is aware of, but there is no object, it is without any factual basis (ex flower of the sky) this vikalpa vritti gives rise to doubtful knowledge.

10 abhava pratyay alambana vritti nidra

The state completely devoid of content or meaning is called as nidra vritti.

11 anubhutavisyasampramosah smrtih

The experience that remains in the mind and not erased totally from it, is called Smrtih

12 abhyasa vairagyabhyam tan nirodah

These five types of vrittis of chitta are dissoluted by practice and detachment.

13 tatra sthitau yatno abhyasah

To stabilise the chitta from practice and detachment, direct the consciousness inwards and constantly practise the eight fold path of yoga with confidence.

14 sa tu dirghakala nairantarya satkara sevito dradha bhumih

This practice should be carried out continuously and for a long time with dedication.

15 drstanusravika visaya vitrsnasya vasikarsamjna vairagyam

State of the consciousness where one is beyond the desire of objects, seen or heard by the sense organs, is known as vasikar samjna vairagyam.

16 tat param purusa khyater gunavaitrsnyam

By param purusa paramatmans darsans or experience the detachment from three gunas rajas, tamas and sattva takes place.

*17 vitarka
vicharanandasmitarupanugamat
samprajnatah*

Vitarka, vichara, ananda and asmita by the relation ship of these the vrittis of consciousness dissolutes; this is known as samprajnatah samadhi or sabijah samadhi.

*18 virama pratyayabhyasa purvah
samskara seso anyah*

When practising continuously. The samskaras diminishes and a yogi experiences only atman and paramatman. This state is known as asamprajnata samadhi or nirbija samadhi.

*19 bhava pratyayo videha
prakrtilayanam*

Videha- beyond bodily attachment and prakrtilaya- beyond prakrti that is panch tan matras namely sabd, sparsa, rupa, rasa and gandha that is word, touch, form, taste and smell and yogis who transcend beyond these, attain bhava pratyaya asamprjnatah samadhi.

20 sraddha virya smrti samadhi prajna purvaka itaresam

By faith, energy, recollection, and intelligence asamprajnatah samadhi is attained.

21 tivra samveganam asanah

An intensive practitioner attains samadhi faster.

22 mrdu madhyadhi matratvat tato api visesah

Mild, medium or strong mode of practice depending on the intensity, the benefits of samadhi derived can be attained faster.

23 isavara pranidhanad va

Or by surrendering to the God, samadhi happens at the fastest.

24 klesa karma vipakasa yair aparamrstah purusavisesa
    isvarah

Avidya and five kleshas, good or bad karma, good or bad results of karmas and desires, one who is untouched by these is regarded as purusavisesa Isvara or GOD.

25 tatra niratisayam sarvajnabijam

He is the ultimate of all the knowledge and there is no boundary for his capacity.

26 *sa esh purvesamapi guruh kalenannvachedat*

That lord cannot be destroyed at any time, so he is the guru of all, the older rishis also.

27 *tasya vachakah pranavah*

One who can say about that lord is pranavah, which is primordial sound AUM.

28 *tajjapastad artha bhavanam*

The japa of Aum should be done with its artha, (meaning) and bhavanam (feeling).

29 *tatah pratyak chetana dhigamo apyantarayabhavas cha*

By doing the japa of that Aum, one gets self realization and obstacles are destroyed.

30 vyadhistyana samsaya pramada alasya virati bhranti
*   darsanalabdha bhumikatva navasthi tatvani*
*   chittavikshepas te antarayah*

Vyadhi, stayana, samsaya, Pramada, alasya and avirati (that is disease, dullness, doubt, carelessness, laziness, loss of interest, delusion and nonattainment of desired objects and unsteadiness) are nine chitta vikshepas or obstacles.

31 dukha daurmanasyamg amejayatva svasa prasvasa vikshepa sahabhuvah

Sorrows, state of mind may be called as boredom, tremors of the body parts and breathing, are factors which contribute to chitta vikshepas or obstacles.

32 tat pratisedhartham eka tattvabhyasah

To remove these vikshepas, abhyasah or practice should be done for ekatattva to know that one lord that is eshwar.

33 matri karuna muditopekshanam sukha dukha punyapunya visayanam bhavanatas chitta prasadanam

Friendship, compassion, cheerfulness towards punyatmas and consideration towards sinners, are the prasadanam of the chitta, when obstacles are removed.

34 pracchardan vidharanabhyam va pranasya

By bringing prana outside by force and holding it, also chitta is calmed down.

35 visayavati va pravrttir utpanna manasah sthiti nibhandhani

Emergence of chitta vritti with divya rupa, divine forms is also responsible for the steadiness of the mind.

36 visoka va jyotismati

Or chitta vritti detached from sorrows, with sattvik light also calms the chitta.

37 vitaraga visayam va chittam

Or detached chitta also becomes steady.

38 svapna nidra jnanalambanam va

By becoming aware about the knowledge of state of dream and sleep, the chitta becomes steady.

39 yathabhimata dhyanad va

Or by meditating on, as per ones interest, which is in any of the chakras or a chosen deity, by this also consciousness can be calmed.

40 paramanu param mahattvanto asya vasikarah

When the obstacles are removed by this, chitta prasad the yogi's perception and control range increases from a particle to a vast sky.

*41 kshinavrtter abhijatasyeva
maner grhitr grahana grahyesu
    tatstha tadanjanata
samapattih*

Just as the transparent jewel gets the same colour of the surface on which it rests, the individual whose vrittis are removed, the clean chitta, atman becomes unified with his innerself and the whole cosmos.

*42 tatra sabdartha jnana vikalpaih
samkirna savitarka
    samapattih*

Samprajnatah samadhi consisting of vikalpas that is sabdha artha and jnana, word, meaning and knowledge as one is known as savitarka samadhi

*43 smrti parisuddhau svarupa
sunyevartha matra nirbhasa
     nirvitarka*

When smriti becomes very pure, within ones own self, the individual experiences void, meaningful silence, known as nirvitarka samadhi.

*44 etayaiva savichara nirvichara
cha sukshmavisaya vyakhyata*

By these savichara and nirvichara one can probe into subtler subjects.

*45 suksmavisayatram chalinga
paryavasanam*

Experiences happening in subtle subjects, in savichara and nirvichara samadhi are beyond the boundaries of time limit.

46 ta eva sabijah samadhi

These samadhis are known as sabijah samadhih.

47 nirvichaara vaisaradye adhyatma prasadah

In nirvichara samadhi after getting enough experience, the yogi gets adhyatma prasadah, gift of adhyatma.

48 ritambhara tatra prajna

At the time when he gets adhyatman prasadah, his buddhi or intellect becomes ritum bhara, the one which can hold the truth.

49 srut anumana prajnabhyamanya visaya vises arthatvat

This ritambhara prajna is beyond sruta, that is vedas, and

anumanajanya prajna, that is generalized knowledge.

50 tajjah samskaro anya samskara pratibandhi

The samskaras, impressions, evolved from ritambhara prajna are capable of removing other samskaras, impressions.

51 tasyapi nirodhe sarvanirodham nirbijah samadhih

When this ritambhara prajnas samskaras are removed, then all samskaras are removed and yogi attains nirbija samadhi.

SADHANA PADA

1   tapah svadhyay esvara pranidhanani kriyayogah

Austerity, self study and surrender to lord, are known as kriya yoga, kriya yoga is a secret technique of life force control, (for further knowledge on kriya yoga refer to AUTOBIOGRAPHY OF A YOGI.)

2   samadhi bhavanarthah klesa tanu karnarthas cha

The kriya yoga is a giver of enlightenment and destroyer of pancha kleshas.

3   avidhya asmita raga dvesa abhinivesah pancha kleshah

Avidhya, asmita, raga, dvesa, and abhiniveshah these are five kleshas.

4   *avidhya kshetram uttaresam prasupta tanuvichinno udaranam*

The kleshas- Prasupta in which kleshas are in a sleeping state, tanu in a subtler state, vichinna in which kleshas are compressed by other kleshas, udara in which they are in action- are evolved from avidhya.

5   *anitya suchi dukhanatmasu nitya suchi sukhatmakhyatir avidhya*

Anitya is to let the mind dwell on the mortal (body) and not on eternity (god). To expect sukha (happiness) from anitya is avidhya (ignorance).

6 *drg darshana saktyor ekatmatevasmita*

Atman and intellect or consciousness, accepting them as one is asmita.

7 *sukhanusayi ragah*

After experiencing sukha, (happiness) what remains as a desire is ragah.

8 *dukhanusayi dvesah*

After experiencing dukha, (unhappiness) what remains as a hate or avoidance is known as dvesah.

9 *svarasavahi viduso api tanvanubhando abhinivesah*

Among the learned ones also, abhinivesah, that is the urge to live further or fear of death remains.

10 Te prati prasava heyah sukshmah

By practising kriya yoga, these kleshas as avidhya, become sukshma − (subtle) and at nirbija samadhi, they return to their original state.

11 dhyana heyastad vrttayah

The enormity of vrittis of these kleshas is destroyed by dhyana.

12 kleshamulah karmasayo dristadristajanma vedaniyah

Karma is initiated by the presense of klesha(s) and karma is rewarded by result (good or bad) and one has to face the result of one's karma.

13 sati mule tad vipako jatyayur bhogah

Till the time the mool or the root of kleshas is there, the karmic cycle of births goes on.

14 te hlada paritapaphalah punyapunya hetutvat

Due to good and bad karmas they give happiness and sorrows as a result.

15 parinama taap samskara dukhair gunavrtti virodha cha
*   duhkham eva sarva vivekinah*

Parinam, taap, and samskara dukh these are resulting, intensive and inborn tendency of sorrows, have conflict with the three gunas sattva, rajas and tamas because of these reasons for the learned individual all karma phallas, results of karmas are dukha rupa, in the form of sorrows.

16 heyam duhkham anagatam

To avoid the suffering that has not yet come, one should refrain from performing such karmas.

17 drastrodrsyayoh samyogo heya hetuh

The blending of the Drasta-(jivatmas) with the drasya, (the nature), is the reason for dukh, which can be avoided.

18 prakasa kriya sthiti silam bhutendriyatmakam
bhogapavargartham drsyam

Prakasa- sattva, kriya- rajas, sthiti-(tamas), is its nature, pancha bhutas earth, fire, water, air, ether, gross sense organs and subtle are its forms, it is for the fulfilment of the beings, that is drshyam or shrusti or nature.

19

vishesavishesalingamatralingan i guna parvani

The five elements (earth, water, fire, air, and ether), the five jnanendriyas, the five karmaendryas and mana form the sixteen tattvas which collectively constitute vishesa. The five tan matras (sparsha or touch, gandha or smell, rupa or form, rasa or taste and sabdha or word) ahamkar or egos are the six avishesas which together with the sixteen vishesas constitute the twentytwo tattvas collectively known as linga. The existence of the lingas is governed by buddhi and prakriti. All these twenty four tattvas take shape from the three gunas (sattva, rajas, tamas) & in the ultimate analysis they are nothing but illusion - maya.

20 *drasta drsimatrah suddho api pratyayanupasyah*

Drasta or jivatman though initially pure, follows the vrittis of buddhi, intellect.

21 *tadartha eva drisyasyatma*

The "drisya", vision Srusti, prakriti or nature is for that jivatman.

22 *kritartham prati nastam apyanastam tadanya sadharanatvat*

This drisya becomes extinct for the one whose bhoga and apvarga work is complete, but it still exists for all others.

23 svasvami saktyoh svarupopalabdhihetuh samyogah

Samyoga is the reason for the existence of Prakrti and purush, nature and soul.

24 tasya hetur avidhya

This relationship between jivatman and prakrti, soul and nature, is due to avidhya.

25 tadabhavat samyogabhavo hanam tad drseh kaivalyam

The absence of avidhya (ignorance) leads to the absence of samyoga (the blending of purusha & prakriti) which destroyes the impressions of past birth and one attains kaivalym.

26 *viveka khyatiraviplava hanopayah*

Viveka jnana, (pure knowledge) which discriminate between avidhya and vidhya, is hanopayah or the way to destroy the hanam or avidhya.

27 *tasya saptadha prantabhumih prajna*

The yogi who achieves the vivekajnana, attains a state of buddhi or intellect which manifests in seven extra ordinary ways.

28 *yoganganusthanad asuddhi ksaye jnanadiptir*
avivekakhyateh

By eight parts of yoga anusthana or practising the asuddhi ksaye happens that is extinction of impurity and by that the light of vivekakhyateh jnana (knowledge) dawns that is the individual sees atman, soul as always separate from body and other attributes.

29 yama niyamasana pranayama pratyahara dharana dhyana samadhayo astavangani

Yama niyama asana pranayama, pratyahara, dharana dhyana and samadhi are the eight parts of yoga.

30 ahimsasatyasteya brahmacharyaparigraha yamah

Ahimsa-(nonvoilence), satya-(truth), asteya-(non stealing), brahmacharya-(non indulgence), aparigraha- (non possessiveness) these are the five yamas.

31 jati desa kala
samayanvacchinnaha
sarvabhauma
   mahavratam

These yamas are not governed by jati-(caste), desa-(place), kala-(time) and hence they are beyond the reason of time, so they are known as mahavratam.

32 saucha samtosa tapah
svadhyayeshvarapranidhanani
   niyamah

Saucha- (internal and external purity), santosa-(contentment), tapah-(austerity), svadhyaya-(self study), eshvara pranidhana-(surrender to lord), are the five niyamah.

33 vitarkabadhane pratipakshabhavanam

When vitarka bhavas, (negative feelings or violent thoughts or unwanted thoughts), gets evolved, then constantly think about their opposites.

34 vitarka himsadayah krtakaritanumodita lobhakrodha moha purvaka mrdu madhyadhimatra duhkhajnananantaphala iti pratipaksha bhavanam

Vitarka- (unwanted tendencies, such as violence) is off three types, krta-(indulgence), karita-(provocation) and anumodita-(abetment or encouragement). The reasons for these are lobha-(greed), krodah-(anger), and moha-(attachment). Their effect may be mild, medium, or strong and sorrows which result infinitely, known as pratipaksha bhavanam.

35 ahimsa pratisthayam tatsamnidhau vairatyagah

When a yogi is established in ahimsa or non violence in his vicinity there is no enemity. He won't have enemity towards any living being; even the wild animals leave their violent nature with such a yogi.

36 satyapratisthayam kriya phalasryatvam

When a yogi is established in satya or non falsehood or truth, his actions become its reward. Things do happen as he says.

37 asteya pratisthayam sarva ratno pasthanam

When a yogi is established in asteya or non stealing, he gets all the wealth.

38 brahmacharya pratisthayam virya labhah

When a yogi is established is brahmacharya or non indulgence, he is benefited by virya or energy.

39 aparigraha sthairye janma kathanta sambodhah

When yogi is established in aparigraha or non possessiveness, he gets knowledge about his past births.

40 sauchat svangajugupsa parairasamsargah

By getting established in external purity, the yogi gets detached from his body parts and he losses the desire to touch others body.

41 sattvasuddhi saumanasyaikagryendriyajayatma darsana yogyatvani cha

Other than above, by getting established in the inner self he becomes pure, which gives rise to cheerfulness, one pointedness, sense control and ability for self realization.

42 santoshadanuttamah sukhlabhah

When one is established is santosh, (contentment), he enjoys incomparable joy.

43 kayendriya siddhir asuddhi ksayat tapasah

By the power of tapah-(austerity), non purity is destroyed and then the body and sense control is obtained.

44 svadhyaya istadevata samprayogah

By svdhyaya or self study one gets his desired goal or istadevata the lord.

45 samadhi siddhir isvar pranidhanat

One gets established in samadhi by surrendering to lord isvara.

46 sthirasukhumasanam

Steady pleasurable pose is asanam or posture.

47 prayatnasaithilya ananta samapattibhyam

When effort ceases, the journey towards infinite begins, in this state of effortless effort the asana is established.

48 tato dvandvanabhighatah

When asana is established, the dvandvas that is duality heat- cold, sorrow-happiness, don't come as obstacles.

49 tasmin sati svasa prasvasayor gativichedah pranayamah

Having accomplished the asana, the interruption in the movement of inspiration and expiration is known as pranayama.

50 bahyabhyantra stambha vrttir desakala samkhyabhih
paridrsto dirghasuksmah

Bahya vrtti-rechak-expiration, abhyantaravrtti- purak-inspiration, stambha vrtti- kumbhak-retention.

Retention may be either between inhaling and exhaling or between exhaling and inhaling, these pranayamas done at desa-place that is heart centre or any other, kala is the time that is for how long, as easy as possible and samkhya that is number. The ratio between inhalation- exhalation and retention may be calculated by some ratio.

51 bahyabhyantara vishayaksepi chaturthah

In sacrificing outer and inner subjects, the pranayama which happens on its own is known as fourth pranayama, that is when breath starts coming out from inside then reverse it and take the breath inside and when it starts coming in, then from inside force it outside and hold it.

52 tatah kshiyate prakasavaranam

There ceasses to exist the avaran or cloud over the prakasha that is vivek jnana.

53 dharanasu cha yogyata manasah

And in dharana mind becomes steady.

54 svavishaya samprayoge chittasvarupanukarah ivendriyanam pratyaharah

While practising pranayama, sense organs shuts off from their subjects and become one with the form of chitta (consciousness) which is named as pratyahara.

55 tatah parama vasyatendriyanam

When pratyaharah is accomplished, senses are controlled in the highest order.

VIBHUTI PADA

1   *desabandhaschittasya dharna*

To bind chitta or consciousness in one place, desa as ajna chakra or sun or moon or any deity is known as dharana.

2   *tatra pratyayaikatanta dhyanam*

In that state of dharana to be aware of an uninterrupted flow of chittavrttis is known as dhyana.

3   *tadevarthamatra nirbhasam svarupasunyam iva samadhi*

When in dhyana, only the awareness of object is there, the practitioners own form diminishes, the chitta becomes a void, then the dhyana, is called samadhi.

4   *trayam ekatra samyamah*

To centre these three dharana, dhyana, and samadhi in one, is known as samyamah

5   *tajjayat prajnalokah*

After accomplishing samyamah one gets alokik knowledge, the knowledge of different planes.

6   *tasya bhumisu viniyogah*

The experience of samyama should be distributed in different stages of chitta.

7   *trayam antarangam purvebhyah*

Trayam-the three dharana dhyana samadhi are inner parts in comparison to yama, niyama, asana, pranayama.

8   *tad api bahirangam nirbijasya*

The above are also outer parts compared to nirbija samadhi.

9   vyuthana nirodha samskarayor abhibhava pradurbhavau
   nirodha ksana chittanvayo nirodha parinamah

In vyuthana state that is emergence state of samskaras, the calming down or dissoluting the samskaras, and in nirodha state, already calmed down state, the samskaras re emerged. This state is the parinama or the result of chitta at the time of nirodha.

10 tatsya prasanta vahita samskarat

By nirodah samskara, the chitta gets steady

11 sarvarthataikagratoyah
ksayodayau chittasya samadhi
*   parinamah*

When vrittis of all subjects of thinking of chitta are destroyed, thereafter only one subject remains; the emergence of that state is the result of samadhi.

12 tatah punah santodiautulya
pratyayau chittasyaikagrata
*   parinamah*

Previously calm and at next moment again emerged, both these vrittis flowing together, this is a result of one pointedness of chitta

13 etana bhutendriyesu dharma
laksana vastha parinama
vyakhyatah

By the result of one pointedness of chitta, one should understand the definition of dharma parinama, religion or natural result, laksanaparinama tendencies as a result, avastha parinama state as a result of pancha bhutas, indriyas, five elements and senses.

14 santoditavyapadesya dharmanupati dharmi

Of Sant-(past), udita-(present) and avyapadesya, (future) the one which remains as a root- support is known as dharmi.

15 kramanyatvam parinamanyatve hetuh

The difference in parinamas is due to time differences.

16 parinamatrayasamyamad
atitanagata jnanam

By doing samyama in the parinamas namely Dharama, lakshana, and avastha, one gets knowledge of past and future.

17 sabdartha pratyayanam
itaretaradhyasatsamkaras tat
*   pravibhaga samyamat sarva*
bhutaruta jnanam

By Practising Sabda-(word), artha-(meaning), rupa-(form) and knowledge, together, a mixed feeling occurs and by doing samyama in their parts, one gets knowledge of languages of all living beings.

18 samskara sakshatkaranat
purvajati jnanam

By samyama when one communes with the samskaras he gets the knowledge of previous incarnation.

19 pratyayasya para chitta jnanam

By communing with others vrtti of chitta he will have the knowledge of the chitta of others.

20 kaya rupa samyamat tad grahya sakti stambhe chaksuh prakasha samprayogeantardhanam

By doing samyama in body form, the acceptance power of the body is withheld, and when the body form is not in contact with thelight of the eyes, yogis body becomes antardhanam, not perceptible to the eyes.

21 sopakramam nirupakramam cha karma tat samyamad
aparanta jnanam aristebhyo va

Sopakram- the karmas that has started producing the effect and nirupakram- the karmas that has not yet started to produce the effect, when one does samyama in these or aristas- the signs of death, he gets knowledge of death.

22 maitryadisu balani

By doing samyama in virtues like friendliness and mercy, one attains their strength.

23 balesu hastibaladini

By doing samyama in elephant and other powerful beings one

gets strength in comparison to them.

24 pravrttyalokanyasat sukshma vyavahita viprakrista jnanam

By doing samyama on subtle planes, vyavahita-hidden treasure and viprakrista-far placed materials, one gets knowledge about these subjects.

25 bhuvana jnanam surye samyamat

by doing samyama on surya or sun one gets knowledge about different lokas or planes.

26 chandra tara vyuha jnanam

By doing samyama on moon one gets knowledge of the position of stars.

27 dhruve tad gati jnanam

By doing samyama on dhruv – pole star one gets knowledge about the motion of the stars.

28 nabhi chakre kaya vyuha jnanam

By doing samyama at nabhi chakra the knowledge, of how the body is made, is attained.

29 kanthakupe kshut pipasa nivrttih

on the throat pit one gets control over urges of hunger and thirst.

30 kurma nadyam sthairyam

By doing it on kurmanadi – one of the nadis vital current passes through the chest region, ones chitta and body become steady.

31 *murdha jyotisi siddha darsanam*

Murdha-brahamarandhara, the jyoti or light in that, is situated in the region of the crown of the head. By doing samyama in this jyoti one gets visions of siddhas, rishis.

32 *pratibhad va sarvam*

By pratibh, knowledge evolved from inner being, the yogi gets insight into everything.

33 *hridaye chitta samvit*

By doing on hridaye- the heart, yogi gets knowledge about chitta consciousness.

34 sattva purusayoratyanta samkirnayoh pratyayaviseso bhogah pararthat svartha

samyamat purusa jnanamBuddhi and jivatman, are separate from each other. To accept them as one is bhoga, this bhoga is parartha, parartha is feeling of separateness from buddhi, by doing samyama in parartha, svartha one gets knowledge of purusa.

35   tatah pratibha sravana vedana darsasvada vartta jayante

By that purusjnana, these six siddhis are obtained pratibh-knowledge evolved from inner being, vedana-tactile power to experience divya touch, or divine touch, adarsa-visual power to see divya rupas or divine forms, vartta-olfactory power, smell power to experience divya gandha or divine smell, asvada-taste, power to experience divine taste divya rasanubhva.

36 te samadhau upasarga vyutthane siddhayah

These above explained siddhis are obstacles for samadhi. They are for the people who are not interested in samadhi.

37 bandha karana saithilyatprachara samvedanacha chittasya para sariravesah

When the reason of binding of chitta ceases to function and prachar-the knowledge of the path. If one have this one can enter into the consciousness and the body of the other.

38 udan jayajjala pamka
kantkadisva samga utkrantis cha

By controlling udana-upward prana, the yogis body doesn't come in contact with water, mire, thorns etc. That is, he gets power to walk without touching either land or water he can walk in air.

39 samana jayaj jvalanam

By controlling samana vayu-prana between the heart and naval area, the body of the yogi becomes fiery and his body shines with a new effulgence.

40 srotrakasayoh sambandha
samyamad divyam srotram

By doing samyama between srotrendriya-sense organs of hearing and akasha-space,one attains the power of hearing divine sound.

41 kayakasayoh sambandha samyamat laghu tula samapat tes chakasha gamanam

By doing samyama in relation with body and space or in light material like cotton, one gets siddhi to fly in space.

42 bahir akalpita vrttir maha videha tatah prakasavarana ksayah

Bahir akalpita-those vrittis of mind- which stay without effort, outside of the body, when the body awareness becomes void. This is also called mahavideha, by evolving of this vritti, the clouding of the brain or avarana gets destroyed.

43 sthula svarupa sukshmanvayarthavattva samyamad bhuta
   jayah

By doing samyama on gross and subtle states of the elements, their essential and all pervading characteristics, and the functioning of their attributes, the yogi gets control over five elements.

44 tato animadi pradurbhavah kaya sampattad dharmanabhi
   ghatas cha

By getting control over these five elements one gets eight siddhis. He attains an excellent body and its functioning becomes unobstructive.

45 *rupa lavanya bala vajra samhananatvani kaya sampat*

Form, grace, dignity and agility like vajra, a weapon with elasticity. These are the treasures of the excellent body.

46 *grahana svarupasmitanvayartha vattvasamyamadindriya jayah*

By doing samyama on the five states of indriyas, (senses) mainly Grahana-(receptivity), svarupa-(nature), asmita-(distinctiveness), anvaya-(attributes), and arthavattva or (purposiveness), with mind, the senses are controlled.

47 tato manojavitvam vikarana bhavah pradhana jayas cha

By that control over senses, one attains the speed in comparison to that of mind, resulting in non dependence on instruments of sense organs, mastery over the nature.

48 sattva purusanyata khyati matrasya sarva bhavadhi sthatrtvam sarvajnatrtvam cha

When one is aware of the distinction between buddhi and purusa, he gets the knowledge and power to deal with all situations of life.

49 tad vairagyad api dosa bija kshaye kaivalyam

When one is detached even from the above siddhis the seeds of the doshas and karmas get destroyed and the experience of kaivalya moksha takes place

50 sthanyupanimantrane samga smaya karanam punar anista prasamgat

In invitation of the people staying near by, one should not involve in their activities, or get attached to them with the feeling of pleasure and pride, by receiving recognition, because by doing these, again you fall into old tendencies

KAIVALYA PADA

1 janmausadhi mantra tapah samadhijah siddhayah

The siddhis   or psychic powers may be obtained by birth, drugs, mantra   or power of words, or by practice of austerities-tapah or samadhi.

2 jatyantara parinamah prakrtyapurat

The transformation from one species to another species is due to the completeness of the nature.

3 nimittam aprayojakam prakrtinam varanabhedas tu tatah ksetrikavat

Good or bad karmas are not the direct cause of the transformation, they act as remover of obstacles to the natural evolution. As farmer who irrigates his fields. Karmas are nimitta, instrumental not upadana in making of an wooden block- the maker is instrumental (nimitta), the wooden block is upadana - so the fundamental changes cannot be brought by human mind.

4   *nirmana chittanyasmita matrat*

The upadana reason of chittas is asmita that is "I"-ness or ahankara, yogi can create chittas by this I-ness.

5   *pravratti bhede prayojakam chittam ekam anekesam*

There is only one chittaa in the midst of seeming manifoldness, this one chitta excites other chittas, towards diversity of activities. Eventhough there may be seeming differences in expressions that is there is worldiness in one and in other the spiritual idealism. Behind them all, there is only one mind, in which there is asmita matra or the sense of "I"-ness.

6 *tatra dhyanajam anasayam*

Among these evolved chittas, the chitta evolved by dhyana is free from desires.

7 *karmasuklakrsnam yaginastrividham itaresam*

Yogi's karma are neither good nor bad, but others karmas are of a three fold good, bad and a mixture of the two.

*8   tatas tad vipaka anuganam
evabhi vyaktir vasananam*

The threefold karmas will give
birth to such tendencies which will
become active   under conditions
favourable to them.

*9   Jati desa kala vyavahitanam
apy anantaryam smrti
      samskarayor ekarupatvat*

In spite of the differences
comming by time, space and
species.There is no difference
between   smriti-memory   and
samskaras. They of identical
nature, so because of our memory
of past tendencies, the chain of
cause and effect is not broken.

*10 tasam anaditvam chasiso
nityatvat*

Since the desire to live has always been present, our tendencies are beginningless.

11 *hetu phalasrayalambanaih samgrhitatvad esam abhave tad abhavah*

It is the motive, which give birth to the accumulated desires. Being dependend and sustained by them and their fulfilment. When they disappear, their motivating factors are removed.

12 *atitanagatam svarupato astyadhvabhedad dharmanam*

There is the time difference between the vrittis of the chitta, and because of this time difference, past and future seems to be different. There is the form and expression we say "past" and the form and expression we say "future" both exist with in the object, at all times.

13 *te vyaktasukshma gunatmanah*

They are either tangible or subtle, according to the nature of the gunas.

14 *parinamaikatvad vastu tattvam*

There is a unity in all things because gunas work together within every change of form and expression.

15 *vastu samye chitta bhedat tayor vibhaktah panthah*

Object being the same, but due to the difference in chitta, different are their panthah-(paths).

16 na chaika chittatantram vastu tadpramanakam kim syat

The object is not dependent on any one of the chittas, because when that object is not the subject of chitta, then what will happen to the object?

17 tad uparagapekshitvac chittasya vastu jnatajnatam

Depending upon the conditioning of the chitta, the object is known or unknown

18 sada jnatas chitta vrattays tat prabhoh purusasyo
 parinamitvat

The swami (lord or jivatman) of that chitta is not parinami- (changeable) that it is unchangeable. That is why, he is always aware of vrittis of chitta.

19   *na tat svabhasam drisyatvat*

The chitta is not self-effulgent, for it is the field, not the knower of the field.

20 *eka samaye chobhayanavadharanam*

Chitta and its subjects, both cannot be known at the same time.

21 *chittantara drsye buddhi buddher atiprasangah smrti*
    samkaras cha

If one chitta is assumed as drsye or scene of the second chitta then the second chitta, has to be assumed as the scene of the other chitta, this will go on infinitely as in a room walled with mirrors. This way the smritis-(memories) will be mixed with each other.

22 chitter pratisamkramayas tad ekarapattau sva buddhi samvedanam

Although jivatman is without activity, detached and changeless, when it comes into the form, it takes the form of the chitta or he gets aware of his chitta.

23 drastri drisyoparakatam chittam sarvartham

Drasta and drisya the observer and the observed, the all pervasiveness of the consciousness in the presence of observer and the observedWhen one realizes the all pervasive nature of observer- observed phenomenon, his chitta becomes aware of all knowledge.

24 tadsamkhyeya vasanabhis chitram api parartham samhatya karitvat

That chitta with innumerable desires and impressions, acts only to serve another atman, for it is a compound combination of different elements, it cannot act independently.

25 visesadarsina atma bhava bhavana vinivrittih

Visesadarsi-one whose perception has a distinctiveness about the difference between chitta and atman, with such a perceptive insight, there is a complete cessation of my-ness.

26 tada vivekanimnam kavalya pragbharam chittam

Then is the mind wisdom oriented, it moves towards liberation.

27 tach chidresu pratyayantarani samskarebhyah

When there are holes or moment of non awareness in the wisdom oriented state. Distraction due to past impression, or recurrence of past tendencies may take place once again.

28 hanam esham klesavad uktam

These may be overcome as done with the kleshas as earlier.

*29 prasamkhyaneapya akusidasya
sarvatha vivekakhayater
    dharma megah samadhih*

Yogi who regards deep meditation not as a means but as an end in itself is endowed with total awareness, arising out of discrimination, since his vivekjnana remains always, he is blessed with dharma megha samadhi or cloud of benediction.

30 tatah klesha karma nivrttih

Then comes the cessation of vrittis of kleshas.

*31 tada sarvavarana malapetasya
jnanasyanantyajjneyam
    alpam*

Then all the knowledge gathered by the mind becomes

utterly insignificant, becomes as nothing in comparisons to that infinite knowledge which is free from all obstruction and impurities.

32 tatah kratarthanam prainama krama samaptir gunanam

Then the sequence of mutations of the gunas comes to an end, for they have fulfilled their purpose.

33 kshana pratiyogi parinamaparanta nirgrahyah kramah

Changes occur only in kshana or instant or moments but they become perceptible in time succession.

34 purusartha sunyanam gunanam pratiprasavah kaivalyam

svarupapratistha va chitti sakter iti

The state effortlessness, where the three gunas no longer have any purpose to serve for the atman, they return to their original state in prakriti. This is absolute freedom or kaivalya. The atman shines in its own nature, as pure consciousness.

qqq

VITAE

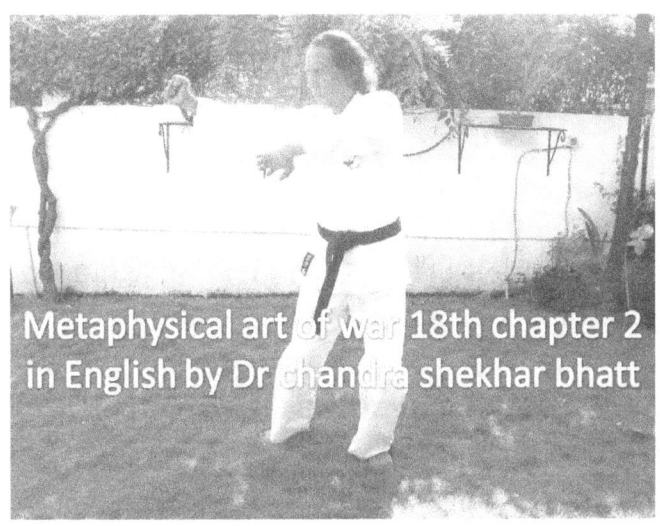

Metaphysical art of war 18th chapter 2
in English by Dr chandra shekhar bhatt

Dr Chandra shekhar Bhatt is PhD in philosophy of alternative medicine from Calcutta. A black belt in shito form of martial arts.Shekhar has named this art Vajramukti which means action to liberation-action in terms of using the techniques of Yoga and martial art that are means to an end- that of controlling mind and body enhancing discipline and nonviolence this fusion has a common objective i.e having a higher level of awareness in life even while searching for absolute truth.

Chronicle Pharmabiz Mumbai

DrChanrashekhar your quantas of philosophical thoughts and in-depth knowledge
of yoga & martial arts has to come in the form of philosophical enquiry who am I.

Dr RAM Bhosle student of Sir Herbert Barker United Kingdom

Dr Chandra Shekhar names his art Vajramukti which means action to liberationaction
in terms of using the techniques of Yoga and Martial arts that are means to
an end...that of controlling mind and body, enhancing discipline and nonviolence.
Indian Express The prestigious Indian newspaper

The modern Indian master Chanreshekhar Bhatt is an exponent of a hybrid of
martial arts and Yoga known as Vajramukti. He has had enough of a following to
Publish books, but you would have to go all the way to Bombay to train with him.   **Shaolin society UnitedKingdom**

Dr Chandra Shekhar has named this art
Vajramukti which means action to
Liberation-action in terms of using the techniques
of Yoga and martial art those are
Means to an end- that of controlling mind and
body enhancing discipline and
Nonviolence this fusion has a common objective
i.e having a higher level of
Awareness in life even while searching for
absolute truth.
Chronicle Pharmabiz Mumbai

www.ingramcontent.com/pod-product-compliance
Lightning Source LLC
Chambersburg PA
CBHW060446290526
45791CB00001B/1